CLAIRE YOUNG

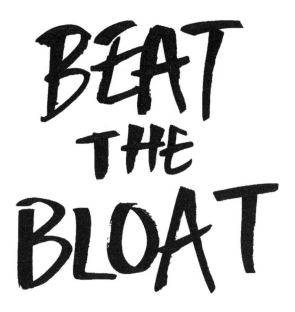

BEAT THE BLOAT

LOSE YOUR BELLY FOR GOOD IN JUST ONE MONTH

This edition first published in Great Britain in 2015 by
Orion
an imprint of the Orion Publishing Group Ltd
Orion House, 5 Upper St Martin's Lane,
London WC2H 9EA

An Hachette UK Company

1 3 5 7 9 10 8 6 4 2

A CIP catalogue record for this book is available from the British Library.

Mass Market Paperback ISBN: 978 1 4091 5827 1

Printed in Great Britain by CPI Group (UK) Ltd, Croydon, CR0 4YY

The Orion Publishing Group's policy is to use papers that are natural,
renewable and recyclable and made from wood grown in sustainable
forests. The logging and manufacturing processes are expected to conform
to the environmental regulations of the country of origin.

Every effort has been made to fulfil requirements with regard to reproducing
copyright material. The author and publisher will be glad to rectify any
omissions at the earliest opportunity.

www.orionbooks.co.uk

Contents

Recipes 87

BEAT THE BLOAT

Introduction

Do you feel sluggish after eating? Do you have a rounded tummy even when dieting? Has your weight-loss stagnated despite calorie counting and healthy eating? Or perhaps there is something 'not quite right' with your digestion?

If you answered 'yes' to some or all of these questions then you've come to the right place.

I've suffered from all of these symptoms in the past and have cured them with a simple diet overhaul. Now I'm slimmer, happier and ready to share my secrets with you.

Do you eat a balanced diet? Or do you actually find yourself eating wheat and sugar in every meal. Perhaps you eat a low-fat diet. But does this really mean that you are overloading your body with carbs and sugar to compensate for the lack of fats and protein?

I truly believe that a real balanced diet means cutting back on carbs so that they no longer dominate your diet. A healthy balance is simply good carbs, filling protein and healthy fats.

I'll show you why you should challenge the conventional wisdom of low fats and high carbs and find a better solution.

If you want weight loss, a flat stomach, healthy digestion and reduced risk of diabetes and heart disease then let me steer you towards the wheat-free revolution.

I challenge you to eat wheat-free for just one month. In 4 weeks, you'll lose weight – up to 4.5kg (10lb) – and it will all come off your tummy. You'll banish food cravings and restore the healthy bacteria in your gut. You'll have taken the first steps towards permanent weight loss, a healthier digestive system and a fitter old age.

Simply banish the bread and unlock the secrets of a flatter stomach.

Yours,

Claire Young, October 2014

Find more recipes, tips and advice at www.beatthebloat.co.uk

1

Beat the bloat

The tummy truth

If you have a fat tummy, love handles or 'man boobs' you are not alone. Look around you. The characteristic paunch is extremely common. It gets worse as you get older, and is virtually impossible to shift through diet and exercise.

But don't despair. There's new and proven thinking that says wheat and sugar are the primary cause of your inflated belly. By updating your diet to avoid wheat and curb your sugar intake you can lose the tum and improve your health prospects.

Why is your tummy so hard to shift? People who are thin and exercise regularly can still have a bulge round their middle. It's also dangerous. The fat that manifests itself superficially in your big tummy is also building up around your internal organs. Your fat tum is an indicator of a fat liver, fat kidneys and a fat heart. This type of fat is called visceral fat and its build-up leads to health complications like heart disease and diabetes. Your thickening waistline tells the doctor that your long-term health is at risk.

Still not convinced? Take a look at an old photo. Before the 1980s people were naturally thinner and healthier. It was in the 1980s that UK health advice changed its focus to 'low fat', starting us on a path to obesity and disease.

Why avoid wheat and sugar?

All carbohydrates, from brown rice to chocolate chip cookies, make your blood sugar rise. Some of the sugar is used directly to provide energy but any excess is converted to fat.

Not all carbs are the same. Starchy or complex carbs such as rice, oats and potatoes release their energy more slowly than sugar, which is a simple carbohydrate. But isn't wheat a complex carbohydrate? Yes. But it has unique properties that actually make it release its energy at the same rate as sugar.

Think how much wheat you eat daily. It's probably part of every meal. And if you have a snack it's likely to be present there too. A diet high in wheat and sugar means that you are building your dangerous fat cells every time you eat. Your body preferentially deposits fat from carbs around your organs and on your belly.

Fat on any other part of your body, from your bottom to your elbow, is not the same as belly fat and is not as dangerous. It is just fat. If you eat more calories than you use for energy, then you will gain fat all over. This is why belly fat is so hard to shift through general diet and exercise. Diet and exercise shift body fat not visceral fat.

Don't blame yourself. You've spent your life being told to avoid fat and eat healthy grains. It's going to be ingrained in your mindset. Just think how your diet is overloaded with wheat, high sugar and low fat foods. Surely this isn't a balanced diet?

A balanced diet is good carbs, protein and healthy fats. Simple.

Lower carbs; higher protein and fats

This diet isn't about cutting out carbs in an Atkins-style diet. Very low-carb diets force your body to produce extreme reactions, not suitable in the long-term.

Instead the diet will be focusing on good and truly complex carbohydrates such as rice and beans, which are digested slowly. Slower digestion means no sugar rush and no visceral fat deposition.

Instead of the empty calories from wheat, we can gain more positive energy from protein and fat. Yes, eating fat doesn't make you fat. It is a rich source of energy and fills you up.

Simple sugars are not cut out entirely. If you cut sugar completely from your diet you are going to crave it and your chances of sticking to the diet are much reduced. Sugar in its more natural forms is the healthiest as it contains vitamins and fibre. Fresh fruits and unsweetened dairy products are a good source of natural sugar.

Bloating

What if the problem is not just a thick waist and a fat tum? If you find yourself sensitive to certain foods, or suffering from wind, bloating or abdominal pain, then your digestive system is under stress.

Food intolerances take many forms and vary hugely in severity. The root cause is undoubtedly genetic. But the number of people with gut sensitivity is growing year on year. Could the problem again be wheat overload? We know that wheat cannot properly be digested and may cause small tears to appear in the intestines.

By cutting out the wheat, understanding our problem foods and restoring gut balance with live cultures, digestive problems start to reduce in intensity and may even be cured entirely.

Food intolerances

Everyone is different when it comes to food intolerances. Some people have to avoid onions, others tomatoes, many others are milk (lactose) intolerant. If you have more severe problems, such as IBS, then you may be intolerant to all of these and more. You may well be genetically predisposed but a lifetime of high-carb foods will have added to the stress on your digestive system. It is likely that if you cut out wheat and take probiotics then you will see an improvement in these symptoms. This may allow you to add them back into your diet, albeit cautiously.

● Milk or lactose

It is very common to be intolerant to the lactose naturally present in cow's milk. This is probably because humans are not genetically predisposed to digest lactose after the age of two. For this reason, lactose intolerance is the least likely to be fixed by wheat removal.

However, lactose-free milk is now common and other dairy foods, notably yoghurt and cheese, contain little or no lactose and can be tolerated unless you are very sensitive.

● Potatoes, tomatoes and aubergines

These seemingly unrelated foods are all part of the same 'deadly nightshade' family and have a similar effect on the gut. So if you are allergic to one of these foods you are likely to be sensitive to the others. Their effect is exacerbated by quantity. You may be able to eat them occasionally with no ill effects but if you eat them often or in conjunction with other digestive stresses, you are more likely to have a bad reaction. If you think these are problem foods for you, cut them out entirely for now, but try reintroducing them slowly at the end of your wheat-free programme. You may be pleasantly surprised to discover that you can tolerate these foods better.

● Onions, garlic and spices

Common 'spicy' vegetables, such as onion and garlic are often considered a trigger point for people with digestive sensitivities or IBS. Depending on your level of sensitivity you may be able to have onion if it is slow-cooked in a stew. Garlic oil is a great way to avoid garlic but still add flavour to your foods. Again, reducing your gut sensitivity by following this programme, may well lead you to greater tolerance and enjoyment of these foods in the future.

The problem with 'gassy' foods

Most starchy carbs release gas during digestion. The superfluous gas in your digestive tract can lead to excessive wind and bloating after eating. The amount of gas produced is dependent on the type of food, with foods such as lentils and beans known for being especially bad. The volume of gas does not vary from person to person, but there is variability in an individual's power to deal with the gas produced. Again, an unhealthy gut will not deal well with the gas. Improving your gut's health through probiotics will mean less bloating and wind with these foods.

If wind or bloating is a particular problem for you, then you should avoid all carbohydrates except rice at the start of your diet. Rice is the only starch that does not produce gas so is the food most likely to be digested cleanly. Removing the wheat and repairing the digestive tract will lead to an increased ability to digest other good carbs. It is important not to cut complex carbohydrates out of your diet completely and to re-introduce them as your gut health improves. The most gaseous foods, like beans, lentils and chickpeas, contain a perfect balance of (very) complex carbohydrate, protein and fibre so are ultimately good for your digestion and your health.

Cut these foods out entirely for 2 weeks while eating wheat-free and taking probiotics. Then try a small quantity of baked beans or similar foodstuff, monitoring your body's reaction. Hopefully you will see only minimal bloating or wind. This should give you the confidence to start adding other complex starches back into your diet.

Hormonal changes

For women, the monthly cycle doesn't start and finish with your period. In the week leading up to your period, and for a few days after, it is common to feel bloated, particularly around the belly. This type of bloating is rooted in the hormones and diet changes only have a minimal effect. The primary cause is a relaxation of muscles in the abdomen. The stomach and muscles around the organs are looser and require more space. This pushes the tummy out. Water retention at the same time exacerbates the problem. It is unfeasible to get rid of the natural process of hormonal bloating, but we can reduce the symptoms somewhat. Lessening the hormonal impact through natural supplements such as evening primrose oil or through high-intensity exercise have been shown to help.

5 life changes for a flatter stomach

1. Cut out wheat entirely

The most important change is to cut wheat out of your diet. As wheat is in so much of the food you eat you'll need to start looking at the packets of every food you buy. Even better, stick to whole, natural foods which don't need a packet and get back to basics with your cooking. Unprocessed fruit, vegetables, meat and cheese are naturally wheat-free.

Avoid

Bread	Crackers	Pancakes
Cake	Pitta or wraps	Breakfast cereals
Biscuits	Beer	Barley
Pastries	Malt or malt extract	Rye
Pies	Pasta	Bulgar
Sausages	Noodles	
(unless gluten-free)		

2. Eat only good carbs

There is a huge variation in how different carbohydrates are digested in the body. Good carbs are digested very slowly and have the least effect on your sugar levels. Note that for some of these carbs, notably rice and potatoes, you need to consume a slightly smaller quantity to reduce your sugar load.

The good carb list

Rice	Quinoa
Oats	Chickpeas
Potatoes	Beans
Butternut squash	Nuts
Lentils	Dark chocolate

3. Eat less sugar

Satisfy your sweetness cravings with fresh fruit, natural yoghurt or dark chocolate. Avoid processed foods containing sugar or sweeteners. Don't drink fruit juices or sugary drinks.

4. Eat more protein and healthy fats

Eat plenty of good-quality protein in the form of chicken, fish and lean red meat. Experiment with eggs cooked in a variety of ways, as eggs contain an excellent balance of protein and fats. Enjoy cheese and fatty meats – but don't go totally overboard. Use olive oil, rapeseed oil or rice bran oil when cooking as these oils have an anti-inflammatory effect on the body.

5. Take probiotics daily

Probiotics are live bio cultures. Think of your gut as a constant battleground between the good and bad bacteria. If you suffer from digestive problems then the bad bacteria may well be winning. The first step to combat this is to reduce the foods that the bad bacteria love to feast on: cheap carbs and sugar, and replace them with prebiotics: resistant starch such as chickpeas and bananas, which is what the good bacterial cultures prefer.

The second, and equally important step, is to reintroduce billions of good bacteria into your gut in the form of probiotics. Choose a quality brand with at least 10 billion bacteria per dose. The more potent probiotics will be more expensive but to have a real effect on the body you need a high dose. Remember you will only need to take the probiotic for a month, as this is long enough to restore a healthy balance of bacteria.

2

Living the diet

Getting started: it's easier than you think

Before you start

- Buy your probiotics in advance. It's important that you start to take them from day one.

- Make your own plan and stick it on your fridge. Use the 5 Life Changes (page 8) as your starting point. Take inspiration from my personal plan in My Food Journal (page 21) and then make it your own.

- Think about what you're going to eat in the first week. Make sure you buy the necessary ingredients so you don't get caught out.

- Remove or throw away any banned foodstuffs from your cupboards and fridge. If you need to keep prohibited food in the house for other members of your family, banish these foods to a separate cupboard and make it out of bounds.

New breakfast routine

It is very likely that your current breakfast contains either toast or cereal so you will need to make some changes. Skipping breakfast is not an option as this will leave you open to temptation later in the day. Don't feel bereft; now is the time to discover a new type of filling and delicious breakfast.

EGGS

Omelette, scrambled or poached – they're all good. Eggs are quick to cook and infinitely versatile. You can add more protein in the form of ham, smoked salmon or cheese. Spring onions, tomatoes or herbs balance the eggs nicely, either combined with the eggs or on the side. It is perfectly acceptable to have eggs every day for breakfast, or try alternating with porridge or yoghurt.

PORRIDGE OR OAT-BASED CEREAL

Oats make a great breakfast as the complex carbohydrates and fibre really keep you full until lunch. Porridge is a great winter warmer and can be made with whole milk or a combination of milk, cream and water. An oat-based cereal, such as granola or muesli, is also good, just check that it is truly wheat-free.

YOGHURT

Full fat natural yoghurt is sweet and filling, and can be combined with oats or fruit to make an even more substantial breakfast. Take a look at Top 5 Ways to Enjoy Your Daily Yoghurt (page 20) for more ideas.

Lunch alternatives

A little advance preparation is needed to make sure you get a filling and healthy lunch. Most of us automatically choose a sandwich, either home-made or packaged, for an easy lunchtime fix. Yet there is a huge range of alternatives out there. The big sandwich chains all offer healthy wheat-free options. Sushi or a salad could be an excellent, if expensive, pre-packaged choice.

By making your own lunch you can open up the options even more. If you want something hot, then soup is a good choice. Lots of vegetables, beans and lentils will make it even more filling. A home-made Tupperware lunch can be substantial and delicious. Making a batch could provide you with lunches for the whole week. Another option is to make an extra portion at dinner the night before.

The simplest and most versatile option of all is to make a salad. Don't think of this as the boring option, there are so many things you can add to make it filling and different everyday.

Salad 101: How to jazz up your salad

THE MAIN EVENT

Cheese: Cheese is often the 'I can't have that' ingredient, but in a salad without bread you can and you should. You want about 40–50g for a main meal. Try feta, grilled halloumi or blue cheese if you want something a bit different.

Meat and fish: As with the cheese, the more flavour the better and if that means something a bit fatty then that's okay too. You need a portion size of about 40g. Thinly sliced chorizo, quick-fried and tossed over a salad tastes amazing. Also worth a try are Polish kabanos, the punchy saltiness of anchovies or some omega-3 rich mackerel. Don't forget thick sliced ham and tinned tuna are excellent standbys.

Eggs: A soft-boiled egg, still warm and quartered on top of the salad will turn it into an event. I boil the egg for 8–10 minutes, run it under the cold tap and peel it as soon as I dare.

SALAD ADDITIONS

Salads needn't be boring. Stock up your cupboard with a selection of flavoursome additions and you can have a different salad every day of the week.

Sunflower seeds: Add bite and protein to your salad by toasting a handful of sunflower seeds in a dry pan.

Roasted red peppers in a jar: Easily located in most super-markets, these add sweetness and flavour to your salad.

Green or black olives: You only need a few so get some top quality olives to make a meal out of any salad.

Sweet piquante peppers: Also known as Peppadew, these come in mild or hot varieties.

Cornichons: These petite gherkins can be added whole to any salad. They go particularly well with ham or sausages.

Pine nuts: Either lightly toasted or just thrown in as they are, pine nuts will add texture and flavour.

A different kind of leaf: Try watercress, rosso, frisée, radicchio or simply a bag of mixed baby leaves.

Houmous: A dollop of houmous really adds flavour.

Walnuts: A handful of walnuts is a great topping, particularly on a salad made with a salty cheese such as blue cheese or feta.

Ready-to-eat puy lentils: Add texture, flavour and filling carbohydrates.

DRESSING

A little dressing brings the whole salad together. Don't go for store-bought 'low fat' (and high sugar) dressings. A drizzle of olive oil and a dash of balsamic vinegar is all you need. Try a chilli- or garlic-infused oil for extra flavour. My recipe for Balsamic Glaze (page 198) adds an extra hint of sweetness without the sugar.

Avoiding wheat

Sometimes you'll need to think outside the box to fill the space on your plate normally occupied by bread or pasta.

CORN TORTILLAS

Tortillas made from pure corn are a great wrap option. They go well with Mexican dishes like fajitas. There are some good corn tortillas out there, but you need to check the label to be assured they are wheat- and gluten-free. All shop bought tortillas are going to contain more ingredients than are ideal but I do like Tortillas Guanajuato from mexgrocer.co.uk, who also sell masa harina, the corn flour needed to make your own tortillas. The best brand I have found is Bfree multigrain wraps, available in a selection of supermarkets.

COURGETTE SPAGHETTI

Courgette spaghetti is a great alternative to pasta. It's quick and easy to make and very versatile. See page 135 to get the low-down on how to make it.

SHIRATAKI NOODLES

These noodles are totally natural and wheat/carbohydrate free. Also called konjac or konnyaku noodles, they are prepared from Japanese yams. These noodles work great in a stir-fry or a Pad thai. Simply rinse in warm water and dry fry for 5 minutes to cook. Shirataki noodles can be bought from Chinese supermarkets or large health food shops.

CAULIFLOWER COUSCOUS

Add substance and texture to your meal with this couscous alternative. Simply blitz the cauliflower in a food processor until you get fine grains, similar in size to couscous itself. Place in a microwave-safe bowl with a little water, a pinch of salt and half a teaspoon of cumin seeds (optional). Cover and microwave on high for 4–5 minutes, or until tender with a little bite.

Food swaps: top 10 guilt-free trades

When you get a craving for these naughty foods, look for the tasty and guilt-free swap.

	Naughty food	*Guilt-free swap*
1	Bread, pitta and wraps	Corn tortillas
2	Chips	New potatoes
3	Crackers	Oatcakes
4	Crisps	Peanuts or cashews
5	Fruit juice	Diluted elderflower cordial
6	Sugary cereal with milk	Granola with yoghurt
7	Biscuits	Dark chocolate
8	Sweets	Grapes or blueberries
9	Ice cream	Home-made low-sugar ice cream
10	Apple pie	Crumble with a ground almond topping

Eating good carbs

Choosing the right carbs, like rice and oats, is key to getting a good balance in your diet. Your body and brain use the slow-release carbohydrates to provide energy. Some good carbs can be eaten in abundance, like chickpeas, but with others, such as rice, you will need to eat less. You can make rice go a lot further by adding extra vegetables such as onions, spinach and peas.

TOP 5 HEALTHY SNACKS

- Cheesy oatcakes
- Nuts such as pistachios or cashews
- Babybel cheese
- Small bowl of olives
- Bowl of frozen berry 'sweets'

Eat more protein and healthy fats

Try and have some protein in every meal. Remember that as well as meat and eggs, protein can also be found in yoghurt, cheese and beans.

Chicken and fish are excellent sources of lean protein, so you can eat as much as you like of these. Red meat, in particularly lean beef, is also a great source of protein and fat. Limit red meat to three times a week as you want to balance saturated fat with other fat sources.

For meat eaters and vegetarians alike, don't forget that some plants contain both protein and carbohydrates. Lentils, beans, chickpeas and quinoa are so perfectly balanced that you can eat as much of these foodstuffs as you like. Get experimenting and try the following recipes: Chorizo and Bean Stew (page 118), Mini

Falafel Burgers (page 188) or Lentil and Mushroom Bolognaise (page 155).

Cutting down on sugar

FRESH FRUIT

Fresh whole fruit offers a little bit of sweetness without the guilt. In fruit, the sugar is offset by water, fibre and antioxidants. Berries are particularly good as they don't have too much sugar and have lots of fibre. Blueberries and strawberries are great when you need a little something after a meal. And don't forget the humble apple.

Bananas are higher in sugar than other fruits, so avoid snacking on them too often. They are useful to provide an energy boost before or after exercise.

YOGHURT

Yoghurt is amazing. It's filling, slightly sweet and delicious. Try a full-fat natural yoghurt. You won't believe how good it tastes and how filling it is. If you like it a little sweeter, try adding half a teaspoon of stevia. The yoghurt completely masks any flavour of the stevia and it just tastes naturally sweeter.

Top 5 ways to enjoy your daily yoghurt	
Jam and granola	Put a teaspoon of low-sugar jam at the bottom of a small dish. Add a generous portion of natural yoghurt and top with a sprinkling of wheat-free granola.

Just berries	Take a generous handful of frozen mixed berries. Leave to defrost for half an hour and then mush with a fork. Add natural yoghurt and stir in.
Elderflower yoghurt	Elderflower cordial adds a heady sweetness but has less sugar than other sources. Add one teaspoon of elderflower cordial and half a teaspoon of stevia to natural yoghurt.
Classic honey	Add a teaspoon of good-quality clear honey to the yoghurt for a richness that adults and children will love.
Oats and blueberries	Get all your goodness in one bowl. Place a handful of jumbo oats in a bowl and add enough water to just cover them. Stand for a minute or two to allow some of the water to be absorbed. Stir in the yoghurt and top with fresh blueberries.

My food journal

Before I start

I am an apple-shaped serial dieter, totally unable to resist sweet stuff and a glass of wine in the evening. I've got 3 young kids and a workaholic husband so am constantly juggling their needs with mine. Not least with mealtimes and food choices. I am also a health-food enthusiast, chocolate addict, bread lover . . .

Start weight	72kg (11st 5lb)
Tummy size (am)	99cm (39in)
Tummy size (pm)	109cm (43in)

Here are my starting figures. I measured my tummy size by measuring round my body at the widest point. I took two stomach measurements. One at the start of the day before eating and one just after dinner. The difference of 10 centimetres (4 inches) between morning and night shows essentially the bloating that occurs as my body struggles to digest the food.

My complete 10-point plan

Here is my personal 10-point plan that I will be following over the next month. This plan is tailored to me and my foibles. For example, I really like peppermint tea and find that it blunts my appetite, aids digestion and reduces bloating. But it's not essential, it's just a helpful tool for me.

My plan is printed and up on my fridge. I see it and am reminded of my commitment at least 20 times a day.

- **Totally wheat-free**
- **Only good carbs**
- **Probiotic supplements**
- **3 square meals a day**
- **Fruit or yoghurt for dessert**
- **Treat of 3 squares dark chocolate per day**
- **Maximum of 2 red meat meals per week**
- **Cup of peppermint tea after lunch and dinner**
- **Strictly no eating between meals**
- **Up to 4 glasses red wine per week, no other alcohol**

Try making your own plan that's perfect for you. Remember the plan needs to be do-able. Allow yourself a treat or two otherwise you could fall off the wagon. If you think you have some problem foods such as tomatoes or beans, then you should consider removing them from your diet for the time being. Remember to incorporate this into your plan.

Week 1: Taking the plunge

DAY 1

Breakfast	2-egg omelette
	Cup of tea
Mid-morning	Cappuccino
Lunch	Greek salad plate
	Natural yoghurt with blueberries
Dinner	Hot steak fajitas
	2 ginger oat biscuits

Day one starts with the challenge of my first dose of probiotics. Why did no one tell me they were so yucky? I have the powdery kind that you mix into a cold drink or food. I think a tablet would be much easier.

The second hurdle is the omelette. Will it take too much effort in the morning? Will I get a hankering for toast or cereal? I actually found the omelette not too hard to make and I've got a plan to make it even easier tomorrow. Coffee and tea with full cream milk is a revelation after years of 'making do' with skimmed milk. I enjoyed both drinks more.

The other thing I noticed after my eggs was that I didn't need lunch until half past one. Normally I like my lunch early so I think the protein-rich omelette really filled me up.

So far, so good. But by lunchtime I found it harder. I just wanted an easy lunch, a quick sandwich is my standard fare. So I really couldn't be bothered making something from scratch. Everything seemed to take ages. I finally chose the Greek Salad Plate (page 122). It was worth the effort but it did feel like something (i.e. bread) was missing. Afterwards I did feel satisfied and happy with my lunch but I know I'm going to struggle with the faff-factor.

Dinner was the totally delicious Hot Steak Fajitas (page 144). I'll be making that again. I felt satisfied but still fancied something sweet afterwards so I made some Ginger Oat Biscuits (page 232). Again delicious and fulfilled my cravings nicely.

By the evening of day one I felt rather bloated, surely not the point. A quick go with the tape measure confirmed this, my tummy size expanded by 2 inches to 45 inches. I was warned that this might be a side effect of starting the probiotics and that it would only last a few days. I really hope that's the case.

Verdict – day one achieved without really missing the wheat and sugar. Want to be a little bit more organised tomorrow, especially with lunch.

DAY 2

Still felt a bit bloated this morning and wasn't hungry for breakfast at all. I know it's important to have something filling as otherwise I would struggle later in the day. I chose some Bircher Muesli (page 96) as it was lighter than eggs and enjoyed it.

Failed to be totally organised for lunch but had some very quick to prepare Smoked Salmon and Cream Cheese on Oatcakes (page 130). Sausage Hotpot (page 175) for dinner.

DAY 3

Weight and tummy size unchanged but feeling less bloated.

DAY 4

Felt very positive and healthy. Saying no to wheat means that there are clear rules on what to avoid which is really helpful. Those biscuits looking tempting in the tin: just say no. A slice of chocolate cake: just say no. I can honestly say that I don't crave wheat, but I do crave sweetness. I know that I can have some fruit or yoghurt, which are both naturally sweet. I am also allowed dark chocolate and it tastes so good.

DAYS 5–7

Enjoyed a quiet and healthy weekend with just a glass or two of red wine as a treat. Unsurprisingly I felt clear-headed and got loads done. I stuck to the rules but enjoyed some really nice meals with the family. By ruling out bread and pasta I was forced to be more creative in my cooking. I found myself making more adventurous meals, such as moussaka, which we all really enjoyed.

I love the fact that I'm still really enjoying food and not feeling in any way deprived. I definitely don't feel so bloated after a meal and feel healthily satisfied.

WEEK 1 RESULTS

Weight	70.3kg (11st 1lb)	1.8kg (4lb) lost
Tummy size (am)	96.5cm (38in)	2.5cm (1in) lost
Tummy size (pm)	104cm (41in)	5cm (2in) lost – difference of 8cm (3in)

Week 2: Getting used to wheat-free eating

Wow! I can't believe I have lost 4lb in one week. Cutting out the wheat is definitely working. Also, I feel the drop in tummy size in the evening is significant. It proves that I am less bloated after eating. My tummy definitely feels less swollen after food.

So week two is about being a stickler for the rules. In week one I felt that I allowed myself a few too many snacks and treats. On one occasion I had quite a lot more than 3 squares of chocolate. I compensated for the lack of wheat by eating more sweet food. I think I'm getting used to wheat-free eating now and need to remember that I also need to stick to good carbs and low sugar.

I have to report that the probiotics have got no less yucky, although I am slowly getting used to them.

Mid-week I discovered sugar-free butterscotch sweets from Marks and Spencer. These were delicious, and I thought, guilt-free. They also satisfied my sweet tooth. However, more than two and I felt it in my gut, a common side effect of maltitol, a sugar alcohol based sweetener (see page 36 for more information on sweeteners). Lesson learned.

WEEK 2 RESULTS

	Current	Change since last week	Overall change
Weight	69kg (10st 12lb)	1.3kg (3lb) lost	3kg (7lb) lost
Tummy size (am)	93cm (36½in)	4cm (1½in) lost	6cm (2½in) lost
Tummy size (pm)	98cm (38½in)	6cm (2½in) lost	11.5cm (4½in) lost – difference of 5cm (2in)

Week 3: Enjoying the wheat-free life

Oh my word! I've lost half a stone. I can hardly believe it. You can really see that my stomach has shrunk and I've been complimented on my changing figure and weight loss.

I've made progress with the probiotics. I am now mixing them with milk and making sure they are fully dissolved before drinking. There's nothing worse than weird powdery lumps left at the bottom of your glass! Drinking the probiotics in milk makes them much more bearable for me, I can hardly taste them now. The probiotics have started to have the desired effect. My temporary bloating and stomach tightening after eating has eased and my weight has fluctuated far less during the day.

WEEK 3: DAY 3

This was the first real challenge of the diet: going out for a curry with friends. I've been a bit worried about alcohol and beer on my night out. I'd normally have a cold beer with a curry: totally out of bounds. Also, would I be able to resist the poppadoms and naan bread?

In the end the evening was so much fun. I felt no guilt as I followed the diet rules perfectly. I also had a surprising revelation. Eating a wheat-free diet is different to other diets. There is no shame or embarrassment in saying that you don't eat wheat. I was able to tell people that I wasn't eating wheat, so avoiding the poppadoms was easy. I had a delicious prawn curry with rice. It was a lovely evening during which I totally forgot about the diet . . . but still stuck to the rules.

It's too early to say for sure but I've started to notice other health benefits too. I normally suffer from a mild form of eczema. This affects my inner elbows and knees and, most annoyingly, my face. But recently I've been able to stop applying the cream and my face is looking so much clearer. This is no coincidence, my skin hasn't felt this soft in years.

I can also suffer from debilitating migraines, which totally wipe me out for a day or two. I haven't had one since starting this diet and I feel less susceptible.

WEEK 3 RESULTS

	Current	Change since last week	Overall change
Weight	68.5kg (10st 11lb)	0.5kg (1lb) lost	3.5kg (8lb) lost
Tummy size (am)	93cm (36½in)	No change	6cm (2½in) lost
Tummy size (pm)	98cm (38½in)	No change	Difference now just 5cm (2in)

Week 4: Thinking about the future

I was a little bit disappointed when I stepped on the scales. Only one pound lost this week. But thinking about what I have achieved already, I know that I can't continue to lose weight so rapidly. This is not a fad diet where I lose loads of weight quickly, only to put it back on again as soon as I stop. It's a long-term plan to make my diet healthier and any weight loss should be permanent.

Looking back to week one and I notice how much my relationship with food has changed in three short weeks. The real and most awesome change is my food cravings and need to eat between meals. I think it took at least a week to get rid of the highs and lows associated with a high wheat intake. After lunch or dinner, which already included fruit or yoghurt, I would still really want a sweet biscuit. My sweet tooth strikes again. Here's the difference. Now I have a filling and substantial dinner with meat or fish and a small quantity of good carbs. I follow that with a cup of peppermint tea. I feel replete and don't think about food again until the next mealtime. This has never happened to me before. I feel healthier and have lost a tremendous amount of weight.

WEEK 4 RESULTS

	Current	Change since last week	Overall change
Weight	67.5kg (10st 9lb)	1kg (2lb) lost	4.5kg (10lb) lost
Tummy size (am)	91cm (36in)	1.5cm (½in) lost	6cm (2½in) lost
Tummy size (pm)	94cm (37in)	4cm (1½in) lost	15cm (6in) lost

The end of my challenge

So the final results are in and I've lost 10lbs in weight. I am ecstatic. I can see that most of the weight has shifted from my tummy. My figure only minimally changes between morning and night. I can see major improvements in my digestive health and bloating too.

Exactly four weeks ago I started my wheat-free challenge. The weight-loss results have exceeded all my expectations. I know I look good and feel tremendous. Although I've still got some weight to lose I am confident that this is achievable.

Impressively, all the weight seems to have come off my tummy. I can clearly see the difference and so can my friends. Tummy weight has always been the most impossible to shift, but mine is now dwindling fast. I know that my tummy was actually the worst kind of fat, visceral fat, that was coating my internal organs and pushing my belly out. I feel tremendously proud of myself and reassured that I'm doing my best to preserve my health into old age.

Into the future

I feel like I've found the key to shifting tummy fat and losing weight. It's hard to believe that the primary factor was my 'daily bread'.

Although I don't feel the need to continue with probiotics, I am still enjoying creamy natural yoghurt everyday. My digestion seems a lot healthier now. I think the probiotics have had a big impact on my ability to digest certain foods. Beans and lentils that previously would have made me bloated and gassy, now have minimal consequence to my weight and tummy size. I used to get a taut tummy after some foods, which felt almost like a balloon to be popped. This no longer happens and my weight and tummy size barely seems to change during the day.

I'm not saying I will never eat wheat again, but I can't see myself going back to it on a daily basis. Perhaps on really special occasions. An artisanal bread roll when I go out for a fancy dinner perhaps. Or my friend's amazing chocolate brownies that she's made especially for me. But not everyday and definitely not shop-bought. I find it so easy now to turn away from the bakery treats at my local coffee shop. Also I have stopped 'borrowing' from the kids' treat cupboard.

Finally, I need to mention the other health benefits of wheat-free living. I haven't had a migraine during the whole challenge and I feel less at risk. Also, my eczema has diminished to such an extent that I haven't needed any creams for the last two weeks of the challenge. My eczema has always been particularly bad around my eyes, making it impossible to wear eye make-up without suffering for several days of red itchy eyelids. This has now changed and I am now free to wear mascara everyday if I wish. For a woman like me in her late thirties, trying to look my best, a little bit of make-up is very important to my self-esteem.

The effects on my eczema and migraines alone are enough for me to avoid wheat. No more debilitating migraines or red puffy eyes. This means so much to me.

If you are still in any doubt about trying the wheat-free challenge and giving up wheat for just one month, please, please go for it. It's made so many positive changes to my life. It starts with dramatic weight loss and a shrinking tummy. But ultimately I've also ended up with a healthier digestion, far, far less bloating, and a totally unexpected improvement in my chronic conditions of migraines and eczema.

Top 10 questions

How much weight can I lose?

When you first give up wheat the weight loss can be quite dramatic. As much as one pound a day in the first week. The rate of weight loss is obviously dependent on how much weight you have to lose, but you should expect upwards of 3 pounds in the first week. After this, the weight loss will settle down but you should continue to lose weight at a rate of 1–3 pounds a week. This diet is not a 'fad' diet, the weight loss is real and permanent.

Why does bloating increase when I start eating wheat-free?

This does not happen to everyone. But a significant number do notice excess bloating as they start the diet. This is primarily due to the probiotics. The probiotics are starting to digest the food properly in your gut. This may mean that more gas is produced at the start, leading to more bloating. When you've been taking them for a short while, you'll see a marked improvement in your digestion. For the first time your problem carbohydrates are being completely digested. The increase in bloating will stop in 3–7 days. After a month of taking daily probiotics you'll notice that bloating, wind and gut intolerances are much improved.

Is eating wheat-free safe in the long-term?

Yes, absolutely. There is no magic ingredient in wheat that your body will miss if you cut it out forever. A diet without wheat is more balanced than one that includes it. Once you've made the changes and got a new wheat-free routine, you'll find that you have no desire to go back to wheat; at least not in the quantities you used to embrace it. By sticking to wheat-free after the initial month of the challenge, you'll continue to lose weight and keep your gut health in check.

What about eating wheat occasionally?

During the month-long challenge you should avoid wheat absolutely with no exceptions. After this period it's up to you. If you think you have been suffering from an intolerance to wheat or gluten then it is likely that you will want to continue to remove wheat from your diet. If your gut health has improved significantly and you don't consider wheat to be a primary trigger for gut problems, you may find that occasional wheat products can be eaten with no negative response. If you do go down this route, be careful to limit your wheat intake and don't let it creep up over time. The problem with adding wheat back into your diet is that if you have it once or twice with no ill effects, you may start eating it more and more. Suddenly you're back to eating it every day and then with every meal. You'll gain weight and your gut health will slowly deteriorate. Set yourself a limit of only one or two portions of wheat a week. Don't just eat some white bread, save your wheat for something really special – some artisan bread or a home-made cake for example.

Gluten-free products – good or bad?

You need to approach gluten-free food products with caution. These processed foods are often full of very quick release carbohydrates such as rice flour and sugar. Your best bet is to prepare your own food, which you can guarantee as gluten-free naturally. However, there are a few food items where you can use the gluten-free guidance to make sure they are suitable.

Good gluten-free foods	Gluten-free foods to avoid
Sausages	Bread
Oat cereals such as granola	Pasta
Oatcakes	Cakes
	Biscuits

Can I really not drink beer?

For some people the thought of giving up beer is more frightening than any other aspect of wheat-free living. But beer contains barley, a form of wheat, and must not play a part in your new diet. The commonly seen beer belly is in fact one and the same as the dreaded 'wheat tummy'.

What about wine and spirits?

The good news is that wine, spirits and any alcoholic drinks that are wheat-free are allowed. Red wine has a positive effect on the metabolism, as it contains antioxidants and other natural anti-inflammatories. Alcohol is digested by the body in a similar fashion to sugar, which is why we need to limit our consumption for weight loss. Don't drink too much in one night as you will get food cravings and are almost guaranteed to break the diet. But one or two glasses of wine or equivalent, up to three times a week is perfectly acceptable.

What exercise should I do while doing the wheat-free challenge?

Exercise is excellent for your general health and mental well-being but it is not the biggest driver for weight loss. I would recommend continuing with your regular exercise routine. An increase of protein and fat in your diet should make exercise easier and more effective. If you don't currently exercise, you should think about adding a fitness programme into your weekly routine. A short walk three times a week is enough to get started. Adding exercise will improve your overall health and help to banish sugar cravings. If you're feeling a little more daring, the back-to-basics running programme known as 'Couch to 5k' is a great way to get started with running. It's free and very simple to start, just search for 'Couch to 5k' online. There are various free smartphone apps available to track your progress. I did it last year, and from a starting point of never running at all, I now regularly run 5k. It's a great way to exercise and gives you a real sense of achievement.

What about fruit juice?

Fruit juice has a very high percentage of sugar. Even though it is a natural fruit sugar, the juice has been processed so much that all the good bits of the fruit have been removed. Drinking fruit juice has exactly the same impact on your body as a sugary drink: it makes your blood sugar rocket. I would recommend removing all fruit juice and sweetened drinks from your diet. Water – still or sparkling – should be your first choice. Coffee and tea are both fine as are all fruit and herbal teas; peppermint tea is particularly refreshing. If you're really craving a fruit juice replacement as part of your morning routine, try a vitamin drink like Berocca.

Artificial sweeteners

Artificial sweeteners, and products made from them, do not have an impact on your sugar levels so are broadly acceptable. However, they are chemical products and can have risks and side effects. Of the artificial sweeteners, the sugar alcohols, such as xylitol and maltitol, are growing in popularity because they are seen to have fewer side effects and to be the most similar to sugar. The problem with sugar alcohols is they are known to upset your stomach. If your stomach is sensitive, even a small dose can cause problems. Erythritol is another sugar alcohol, which is more completely absorbed than others, so is less likely to cause digestive disturbance.

You should find your need for sweetness, either sugar or artificial, will reduce markedly as you gain control of your blood sugar levels. If you want to sweeten foods without sugar, the natural zero calorie sweetener, stevia, should be your first port of call.

3

The relationship between your body and what you eat

What's wrong with wheat?

You may think that eating wheat, especially wholegrain wheat, is good for you. You may think that it is impossible to give up all foods containing wheat. I believe that both these assumptions are wrong. I took it for granted that wheat was healthy for my body and that giving up wheat would be hard. I was totally mistaken on both counts.

The wheat epidemic

Why do we think giving up wheat is hard? Because it is in every meal that we eat and every snack that we purchase. Walk down the cereal, snacks or even healthy eating aisles at the supermarket and you would think that wheat and sugar were our only available foodstuffs. 'Low fat' and 'Healthy whole grains' labelling is everywhere. But try finding 'Low sugar' or 'Wheat-free' and you are forced down the special diet aisle.

The nutritional advice offered to us since the 1980s suggests that a low-fat, high-carb diet is the way forward. Recent statistics have shown that there is a direct correlation between the start of this advice in the eighties and nineties and our expanding waistlines, metabolic syndrome and the rise in type 2 diabetes. Latest UK figures* show there were 0.8 million diabetics in 1980 (before the endorsement of a high-carb, low-fat diet), 1.4 million in 1996 and 3 million in 2010. The most recent figures from 2013† stand at 3.2 million diabetics, meaning that the number of diabetics in the UK has quadrupled in 30 years. One in 17 of us (6%) is now diabetic.

Scientific research is at last showing this advice to be detrimental to our health and the news that carb overload can be damaging is finally starting to reach the public's consciousness. But the medical profession is resistant to change and public health advice is still very much of the low-fat variety. Indeed this advice is now so lodged in our brains that eating butter and full-fat milk seems contrary and wrong. Most of us have been educated all our lives that bread, cereal and whole grains are the backbone of a healthy diet and it's going to take time and a change in policy before we start to feel that fat is good and sugar is bad. In the meantime UK retailers will continue to peddle cheap foods loaded with wheat and added sugar as health products.

Modern wheat

The wheat we currently eat is a far cry from that of our ancestors. In fact it is totally different from the wheat we grew and ate just 100 years ago. In the 1940s and 1950s a new agricultural revolution

---

* Diabetes UK. 'Diabetes in the UK 2004', http://www.diabetes.org.uk/Documents/Reports/in_the_UK_2004.doc

† Diabetes UK. 'Diabetes prevalence 2013 (February 2014)', http://www.diabetes.org.uk/About_us/What-we-say/Statistics/Diabetes-prevalence-2013/

was born. With the admirable goal of curbing world hunger, new scientific techniques were developed to dramatically increase wheat yield. New strains of wheat were created that increased yield by a staggering 800%. The new dwarf wheat did indeed help solve world hunger, but it also had some totally unexpected implications.

It was assumed by everyone that as the new wheat remained essentially just 'wheat', there were no health concerns. Wheat is wheat and human health was never considered to be at risk. Yet the gluten structure of modern wheat is dramatically different to that of just 100 years ago. Ancient wheat contained three times more protein than the modern variety. Our bodies have simply not had time to evolve to digest this new wheat effectively.

We now eat so much of this new cheap wheat that we are totally overloaded with a substance that cannot be properly digested. This has huge implications for our health and weight and goes some way towards explaining the huge surge in gluten intolerance and coeliac disease that is currently sweeping the modern world.

Are you intolerant to wheat?

Did you know that up to 50% of us have some intolerance to wheat?

I never believed that I was intolerant to wheat. But since giving it up, my digestion is healthier, my eczema has totally disappeared and I am no longer susceptible to migraines. Eczema and migraines have been a blight on my life since I was a teenager. Although never a serious sufferer of either, countless visits to the doctor and various creams and drugs never touched the root cause and they became an annoyance that I learnt to live with. Three weeks after giving up wheat these chronic problems totally disappeared.

The most common mistake we make is to assume that gluten intolerance just affects our digestion. So if we are not suffering from abdominal pain, bloating or diarrhoea, we think that food cannot be the cause of our ills. In fact over 50% of diagnosed coeliacs do not show the classic symptoms. Instead the new symptoms of the disease include anaemia, skin complaints and allergies. Coeliac disease is on the rise, increasing 400% in the last fifty years, showing a direct correlation with the introduction of new wheat.

If you are not coeliac, could wheat still be affecting you in other ways?

Signs and symptoms of gluten sensitivity

- Anxiety
- Bone pain/osteoporosis
- Brain fog
- Dairy intolerance
- Delayed growth
- Depression
- Digestive problems such as bloating, diarrhoea, constipation, abdominal pain
- Irritable bowel syndrome
- Low immunity
- Nausea and sickness
- Skin complaints such as dermatitis, eczema, hives

The effect of wheat on your immunity

There is a protein in wheat gluten that has the unique ability to damage the walls of the intestines. If your body has been overloaded with wheat for years then the intestinal tract could be fragile. Undesirable bacteria can filter through the torn cell walls and gain entry into the bloodstream, making the body less able to fight common bugs and viruses. It may also trigger the body's autoimmune response, where the body is tricked into attacking healthy organs. This can lead to autoimmune conditions such as thyroiditis and arthritis.

When you give up wheat you allow the gut to rest and repair. Taking probiotics helps the healing process and makes you less susceptible to common illnesses.

Wheat, blood sugar and insulin

Why is wheat so much worse for weight gain than other foods? The process of weight gain starts with high blood sugar. When you have excess sugar in the blood it is converted to fat. Wheat causes the biggest surge in blood sugar of all normal foods. That's higher than pure sugar, higher than a chocolate bar and higher than ·a can of Coke. What's more, this result goes for all kinds of bread. Sliced white, granary and wholemeal all give the same blood sugar surge.

Wheat is, as we all know, a complex carbohydrate. Surely that should make it harder to break down than the simple carbohydrates in sugar? No. Wheat contains the highest proportion of the most easily broken down carbohydrate, called amylopectin A. Wheat is the most volatile of carbohydrates, simple or complex, making it the most digestible foodstuff of all.

This matters because repeated high blood sugar is the first step on the road that leads to obesity and type 2 diabetes. When your blood sugar levels rise, insulin is pumped from the pancreas to move the sugar to where it's needed. The higher the blood sugar, the more insulin is released. When you have regular floods of insulin, your body becomes less sensitive to the insulin signal, so the pancreas releases even more insulin. This is insulin resistance. Insulin productivity can increase until it reaches its maximum peak. If this is still not enough, the result is unmanaged blood sugar, in other words, type 2 diabetes.

Wheat and ageing

The same problem with high blood sugar can lead to an accelerated ageing process. A new marker for biological ageing is proving useful in showing what impact lifestyle choices have on how you age. Advanced Glycation End products (AGE) is the name given to useless waste products that are deposited around the body. The outward effects of AGE could be wrinkles, sagging skin or arthritis. The number of AGEs you have throughout the body increases as you grow older. But if you have more of them than you should for your age, then the ageing process is accelerated.

The higher your blood sugar, the more glucose molecules there are floating around in your body looking for a home. Some of the spare glucose bonds with protein in the body's tissues and organs. Once this bond is formed it is irreversible and the AGE floats around the body, clumping together with other AGEs and causing blockages. These blockages could eventually lead to heart disease, kidney failure and blindness.

It's important to remember that AGEs are a natural function of the ageing process. The danger is that with continually raised blood sugar, more AGEs form and you age quicker.

Wheat and weight loss

Big fat stomach, love handles, man boobs . . . are they caused by wheat? High sugar and a sedentary lifestyle have added to the problem, but the primary cause of continuing weight gain is wheat.

We have already seen that wheat causes a surge in blood sugar and insulin. The rush is higher than essentially any other food. If there is any unused blood sugar, insulin effectively converts the sugar into fat cells. Your blood sugar goes in cycles, rising straight after a high carbohydrate meal and then dropping two hours later, requiring another fix of more bad carbohydrates. So you could easily be depositing fat after every meal and snack, accumulating fat rapidly and depositing it as deep visceral fat around your waist.

WHEAT IS ADDICTIVE

As well as causing an endless series of blood sugar surges and crashes, wheat can trick you into eating more and more. That blood sugar high that you love is actually a rush of exorphins. Exorphins are released when wheat, specifically gluten, is broken down in the stomach. It enters the bloodstream and stimulates the brain's 'happy' or morphine receptor. This is the same receptor that is triggered with naturally produced endorphins when you exercise.

Wheat stands proudly with alcohol and caffeine as being the only foodstuffs that affect the central nervous system. It induces a pleasurable effect that leaves you craving more and more. When you remove wheat from your diet, you may experience mild withdrawal symptoms. The withdrawal symptoms can be easily conquered in less than a week.

WHEAT IS AN APPETITE STIMULANT

Do you feel the need to graze on unhealthy foods after meals, particularly in the evening after dinner? This is a common phenomenon and one to which I admit to being very susceptible. You know that you are not hungry, but can't resist the lure of the biscuit tin. Like an addict, you prowl the kitchen cupboards searching for something to satisfy your ache. The addictive properties of wheat strike again. It stimulates your appetite and spectacularly crushes your willpower. Cutting out the wheat stops this process in its tracks.

What is the most helpful tool that going wheat-free has given me? It's given me willpower and the ability to say 'no' to tempting foods. Cutting out those night-time calories will make you lose weight.

REMOVE THE WHEAT FOR REAL WEIGHT LOSS

If you cut out the wheat, you'll lose weight rapidly. It's as simple as that. A drop of 5 pounds or more in the first week is not uncommon, and weight loss of over a stone during a month is more than possible.

As soon as you break the highs and lows of the blood sugar cycle, the fat build-up halts. You eat only when you're hungry, and your ability to say no to snacks increases dramatically. You are naturally reducing your calorie intake, without feeling deprived. Rapid weight loss is the result, and it will all come off the tyre round your middle.

Good vs. bad carbs

Carbohydrates and blood sugar

Blood sugar is a measure of how much sugar or carbohydrate we have available for energy in our body.

Sugar is a simple carbohydrate; it is converted directly to energy. Other carbohydrates are complex, meaning that they need to be broken down by the body before being turned into energy. Scientists have measured the body's ability to break down foods into sugar and it is this that is used to define what are good and bad carbohydrates.

Sugar highs and lows

We all know what we mean by a sugar high: that brief feeling of sustenance and energy when we've eaten lots of sugary carbohydrates. But do you know it's always followed by a low? Within two hours of eating high-carb foods, we feel a drop in energy and mood followed by a feeling of hunger, rumbly tummy and that inevitable search for more bad food. It's a vicious cycle that many of us are forever fighting against.

When we eat high-sugar foods, energy is released quickly through the body. Unless it is used straight away, by exercising for example, the body sees that energy as excess and does what it thinks is the sensible thing: it stores the energy as fat.

How do we fix it?

Simply stop the highs and lows and occupy a happier, more satisfying middle ground. By eating mainly good carbs, proteins and fats we'll feel full after we eat and for many hours afterwards.

Our overall food consumption will naturally go down and we'll lose weight, particularly that obnoxious belly fat which accumulates as a direct result of our sugary ups and downs.

Practically, we need to stick to good carbohydrates. Bread, pasta and anything made from wheat flour are the worst offenders so cut them out completely. Sugar, particularly added sugar, also needs to be kept to a minimum. Essentially, we need to keep the sugar load on the body low.

The sugar load is the most complete measure of how our bodies digest, absorb and use different carbohydrate foods to provide energy to the body. It uses the scientifically calculated GI value as its basis and then also takes into account the available carbohydrates, the fibre content and portion size.

To keep blood sugar balanced with no peaks and troughs, eat foods with a low GI, low available carbohydrates, high fibre content or a combination of all or any of the above.

Foods that do not contain any carbohydrates such as meat, fish and cheese do not have an impact on blood sugar.

Don't ever think of carbs as bad; they are an essential part of your diet. You just need to reduce the quantity so that they never make up more than a third of your meal.

In fact as a guide it should be 33% good carbs, 33% protein and fat, 33% vegetables and fruit.

The good carb list

Stick to only the carbohydrates on this list and you won't go far wrong.

RICE

Brown rice and basmati rice are both good carbohydrates. Brown rice has more fibre so is slightly better than basmati. The quantity of rice that you eat is important too. Stick to 30g dry weight or 80g cooked weight of rice. This is a smaller amount than the portion size stated on the packet. Try adding veggies such as onions, peppers and peas to your rice. These will add oodles of flavour as well as giving you a hearty portion. There are several simple rice ideas in the Sides and Veggies chapter (pages 191–204).

If you find that the cooking time for brown rice is off-putting, try buying the pouches of pre-steamed rice that go from packet to plate in 2 minutes flat. I like Tilda Brown Basmati rice as it has no unexpected ingredients.

OATS

Oats contain a very special and unique ingredient: beta-glucan. Beta-glucan is a type of fibre that means our bodies digest the carbohydrate more slowly and evenly. Oats therefore release their energy more slowly than other carbs and keep us fuller for longer. Oats are particularly good as a breakfast ingredient as they are so filling. Stick to a portion size of 40g dry weight or less – you won't need more.

Porridge oats are the standard oats we buy for porridge. Be careful to avoid 'quick' or 'express' oats as these have been overly processed with a lot of the goodness removed. Jumbo oats are bigger than porridge oats and have an even lower sugar load. They are also known as whole, traditional or old-fashioned oats and are my preferred choice for all kinds of baking.

Oatcakes are more processed than whole oats but still contain lots of beta-glucan. They make a great snack or light lunch when loaded with your favourite toppings.

Oat bran is the most concentrated form of beta-glucan. It's finely milled and is a great baking ingredient. I buy Mornflake oat bran which you can buy in major supermarkets and health food shops.

POTATOES

Choosing the right sort of potatoes is crucial. New potatoes boiled in their skins and a potato baked in its skin are good carbs. Mashed potato and chips are bad carbs. They key is in the skin, which adds fibre, texture and flavour. A good portion size is 150g – 3-4 new potatoes or a small jacket potato. This means that the all-time winter warmer of jacket potato, baked beans and cheese is a good option – just don't forget to eat the potato skin.

It is possible to be intolerant to potatoes as they are part of the deadly nightshade family, along with tomatoes and aubergines. Intolerance could lead to an increase in bloating or IBS symptoms. If you think this might affect you, then it is best to leave out potatoes from your diet entirely. Don't despair because balancing your digestive system by living wheat-free and taking probiotics could mean that soon you'll be able to eat these versatile vegetables once again.

BUTTERNUT SQUASH

Butternut squash has a much lower impact on blood sugar than similar foods such as sweet potato and pumpkin. It's tasty and naturally sweet and goes really well in a range of vegetarian dishes or as a side dish with meat or fish.

LENTILS

Lentils are an amazing blend of good carbohydrate and protein. They are also extremely versatile. Puy lentils are great in all kinds of stews and salads, adding a unique nutty flavour and texture. Red and brown lentils are used in a lot of Indian cooking. They make a great main vegetarian dish.

QUINOA

Quinoa is another food that mixes carbohydrate and protein. A simple grain without much taste of its own, use it as a meal accompaniment or anywhere you might previously have used couscous.

CHICKPEAS

Chickpeas are the most versatile and well balanced of the foods that mix carbs, fibre and protein. Use them to make falafel or in stews. When baked they make a fine crunchy snack too. Gram (chickpea) flour is made from chickpeas and makes a useful wheat flour substitute in savoury dishes.

BEANS

Kidney beans, cannellini beans – even baked beans – they're all good. If you're buying baked beans, check the ingredients list for too many nasties – look for varieties with reduced sugar and salt.

NUTS OF ALL TYPES

Nuts contain varying amounts of carbohydrates and usually quite a lot of good fat. They are very filling and do not raise your blood sugar by any significant amount. They therefore make a great snack.

DARK CHOCOLATE

Saving the best until last! Dark chocolate (70% cocoa solids) is a really good carbohydrate. It contains some sugary carbs but this is diluted by a good proportion of fibre. Use in cooking or snack on a few squares when you feel a craving.

The bad carb list

The bad carb list contains only four things: bread, pasta, sugar and cakes. Yet unfortunately these foods play a huge part in our everyday diet. Without care and attention they'll be in every meal we eat. If you buy pre-packaged or prepared food, check the ingredients list. Wheat and sugar are in absolutely everything.

BREAD

Bread is top of the bad carb list because it is so easy for the body to convert into sugar. Wholemeal bread increases your blood sugar more than pure sugar does, so two slices of bread is really little different, and often worse, than drinking a can of fizzy drink.

PASTA

Pasta is made from wheat flour but the processing and compression leads to some unique properties. Although blood sugar levels do not rise very much initially, pasta generates high blood sugar levels for up to six hours after consumption. The sugar load of pasta is therefore nearly as high as bread.

SUGAR

Sugar, and anything containing sugar, should be treated with extreme caution. Pure sugar obviously affects your blood sugar almost immediately. But if you cut out sugar from your diet you'll create a diet plan that is impossible to stick to and will leave you primed to gain weight at your earliest failing. Sugar occurring naturally in whole fruits is much better for you as the fruit sugar (fructose) is balanced by dietary fibre. A little bit of sugar goes a long way and I do recommend using small amounts of natural sugar, such as brown sugar and honey, as these add flavour as well as sweetness. I like to blend sugar with naturally sugar-free stevia to get a sweet taste without compromise.

CAKES AND BISCUITS

Cakes and biscuits contain the double whammy of wheat flour and sugar so are notoriously bad. They are also the hardest thing to give up, especially if you have a sweet tooth. It is very difficult to buy cakes and biscuits with no flour or sugar and if you decide to make your own there will be sacrifices to make. I've included some of the best no flour/low sugar recipes in the Baking and Cakes chapter (pages 223–236) so go and experiment. Chew on a square or two of dark chocolate and think that it's not all bad!

Low carbohydrate foods that can be eaten freely

MEAT, FISH, EGGS AND CHEESE

These foods do not contain carbohydrates so do not affect blood sugar. They are made up of proteins and fats and should constitute about a third of most meals. Proteins and fats are the most filling and calorific part of most meals so consideration should be given to the quality and health properties of your chosen foodstuff. See Healthy Fats and Meat, (pages 56–60) to find the best choices for you.

FRUIT AND VEGETABLES

Fruit and vegetables do contain some carbohydrate, often in the form of simple sugars. In vegetables the carbohydrate content is low and is offset by the natural fibre, making a minimal impact on blood sugar.

Fruit obviously contains a bit more sugar than vegetables but should never be avoided as it has other health benefits. Also, most fruits contain enough fibre to dilute the blood sugar effect. Eating the whole fruit, rather than processed, crushed or cooked will always give you the most benefits.

The best fruits are berries, apples, pears and kiwis. All whole or minimally cooked or crushed fruit can be eaten freely. Bananas are an interesting case as they do have a lot more natural sugar than other fruits. Bananas are best saved for extra energy before exercising or as an occasional treat.

Dried fruit has a much higher sugar content so should generally be avoided. It can still be eaten in small quantities and used in cooking.

Milk and yoghurts are similar to fruit, in that they do contain some natural sugars. But eating full-fat milk and natural yoghurt has a minimal impact on blood sugar. Yoghurt also has the major advantage of containing live cultures that aid digestion, reduce bloating and improve gut health.

The sugar impact

Every sweet food that we eat contains a form of sugar. There are three basic building blocks of sugar.

- **Fructose** is found naturally in fruits and honey and is the sweetest carbohydrate.
- **Glucose** is the primary metabolic fuel for the body and is found in all starchy foods.
- **Galactose** is found in dairy products and is converted to glucose by the body.

Other sugars that we eat are combinations of these basic sugars. Table sugar, also known as sucrose, is a mixture of fructose and glucose. The milk sugar lactose is glucose and galactose.

What we think of as 'sugar' is a combination of glucose and fructose. The body deals with these sources in totally different ways.

Glucose is processed by every cell in the body. When we consume glucose, sugar is liberated to our blood and our blood sugar levels rise. If we consume more glucose than our body needs, we produce more insulin which then stores the excess calories as fat. So our bodies need glucose, but not too much. As glucose is not particularly sweet we tend not to crave it as much as fructose.

Fructose, on the other hand, is very, very sweet and anyone with a sweet tooth is addicted to the stuff. Fructose is metabolised by the liver, which is why it does not raise the blood sugar and is said to have a low GI. A little bit of fructose is not a bad thing. It's all about quantities. If you eat more than a small dose of fructose, the liver cannot metabolise it effectively and this triggers an insulin response.

Fruit and honey

Anything that is remotely sweet, with the exception of milk and yoghurt, contains fructose. Fresh fruit contains water and fibre along with the fructose, which will dilute the effect. So the little bit of fructose in fruit is acceptable to our bodies. We can apply the same rules to our cooking to reduce the fructose effect of our food. For example, using a small quantity of honey (which is higher in fructose than table sugar) in our cooking may be acceptable, especially if we balance it out with fibre-rich ingredients like oats or cocoa.

Stevia: naturally sweet

Unfortunately, the quantity of sugar we can consume without overly raising our blood sugar and insulin levels is quite small, which means we have to look at alternatives when we want our fix of sweetness.

There are some people who don't look to sweet food when they are peckish or after a meal, but they are in the minority. Most of us love to finish a meal with something sweet. We also love to snack on sweet foods when we are tired or stressed.

The simplest and safest way to get your sugar hit is in the form of fresh fruit, natural yoghurt or even a few squares of dark chocolate. But sometimes this is not enough and we want a sweet treat. When I want to eat something sweet I often turn to stevia as a natural sweetener. Stevia is not an artificial sweetener as it is derived from a natural source. It does not have the hazards to your health or gut that are sometimes associated with artificial sweetener brands.

The most common form of stevia in the UK is Truvia®. This is a brand name from Silver Spoon and is available in all major supermarkets. Truvia® is by no means perfect, it is processed and contains bulking agents. It also has a noticeable aftertaste if too much is used. But as the only stevia commonly available in the UK, it's the one I use in all my baking and cakes. On the packet it suggests that you need to use approximately one-third of the quantity compared to sugar. In my experience I have found that you should use a little bit less than that. When mixed with chocolate or dairy, no aftertaste is noticeable. Also, vanilla seems to blend beautifully with stevia to make a very natural taste.

When baking, I find a combination of sugar or honey with stevia gives the best flavour, without exceeding sugar tolerance levels. If a recipe suggests 100g caster sugar, I would suggest an equivalent of 15g (1 tbsp) stevia and 15g (1 tbsp) sugar gives a good balance of taste and sweetness. As you can see, you need only a sixth of the sugar and associated calories when you add a little bit of stevia.

Healthy fats and meat

Fat does not make us fat. I know that this feels contrary to every piece of diet advice that you have ever received, but fat is essential for our bodies. Fat fills us up so we don't overeat and is the fuel that our bodies prefer.

Key facts

- Fat on its own is not bad for you. It is a combination of saturated fat and bad carbs that is dangerous to our health.
- We need both saturated and unsaturated fat in our diet.
- Eating cholesterol does not give you high cholesterol.

Let's go back to the start and look at our 'thrifty' gene. This is the gene inherited from our Stone Age ancestors. Before agriculture, our diet was mainly fat and protein from meat and some simple sugars from fruit. There was very little starchy carbohydrate available. This diet is still the preferred choice for your body. The thrifty gene was programmed to store food as fat during times of abundance. Our modern diet is plentiful, so whenever we have excess food this is turned into fat. So the thrifty gene, unchanged since ancient times, genetically favours those with a high disposition to store fat. Every modern human is pre-determined to store fat, ready for a food shortage that does not materialise. Unfortunately we have approximately 50,000 years to wait for our genetics to catch up with our change in diet.

Saturated fat and cholesterol

Saturated fat has for several decades been thought of only with fear. Saturated fat is found naturally in meat, eggs and dairy products. It is the most densely calorific of foodstuffs, which is enough to make any seasoned dieter remove it from their diet as much as is humanly possible. Yet it is a natural product, chock full of essential vitamins and fatty acids. And the very fact that it is high in calories is what makes it good for you. It fills you up, making you satisfied and unlikely to overeat. Increased intake of fat will decrease your need for carbohydrate. So eating fat is going to make you eat less, not more.

All foods containing saturated animal fat contain cholesterol. This means meat and particularly eggs are high in cholesterol. But the cholesterol that we eat is different from the one produced by our bodies. The one found in foodstuffs is not readily absorbed, so eating a source of cholesterol does not have a significant impact on the concentration of cholesterol in the blood. Conversely it has now been found that carbohydrates actually increase the level of LDL (or 'bad') cholesterol in our bodies, the one that thickens the arteries and eventually leads to heart disease.

Carbohydrates and saturated fat together is by far the worst combination, as this does lead to raised levels of cholesterol. Hence why a burger in a bun is really bad for you but a home-made burger with a salad is an excellent meal.

Unsaturated fat

Unsaturated fat is also necessary in our diet. Some of it is good for us and some not so good. As a general rule, the healthiest fats are the most natural and least processed fats.

MONOUNSATURATED FAT

Monounsaturated fat, also known as omega-9, has a positive effect on your health. Monounsaturated fat is good for your heart. It can have a positive impact on cholesterol levels and helps reduce clogging in the arteries. Olive oil and rapeseed oil are rich sources of omega-9.

POLYUNSATURATED FAT

Polyunsaturated fat can be split into omega-3 and omega-6 fats, which have very different properties.

Omega-3 is the good polyunsaturated fat. Omega-3 has an anti-inflammatory effect on the body, reducing the risk of all manner of diseases. The richest natural source of omega-3 is fish, especially salmon and pollock. Eating fish at least once or twice a week provides good-quality protein and omega-3s, which is good for our heart as well as our weight. Omega-3 is also present in red meat, particularly beef. All British beef is naturally grass-fed which makes it an excellent source of protein, saturated fat and omega-3.

Omega-6 is the bad polyunsaturated fat. Omega-6 has an inflammatory effect on the body. If your diet is laden with omega-6, with very little omega-3, this can increase the risk to your heart and brain as you age. Sources of omega-6 are not natural products. They are highly processed oils and, unlike olive oil and butter, are relatively recent additions to our diet. The technology needed to prepare these oils has only been invented in the last 50 years. Oils loaded with omega-6 include vegetable oil, sunflower oil, groundnut oil and corn oil.

Most oils and fats include a mix of saturated and unsaturated fat. All three forms of unsaturated fat are likely to be present. It is the ratio of good to bad fats that determines the health-giving properties of the oil. Saturated fat is good as long as it is not combined with bad carbohydrates. Monounsaturated fat and omega-3s are also good, whereas the proportion of omega-6 fats should be kept to a minimum.

The best fats for cooking

The oils we have in our cupboards may not be as good for us as we first thought. For many years we have been encouraged to consume polyunsaturated oils such as sunflower and vegetable oil. These are the ones with the highest proportion of omega-6. Instead the first oil you should reach for in cooking is olive oil. If this is unsuitable due to its flavour or relatively low burn point, rice bran oil or rapeseed oil are the best oils to use.

OLIVE OIL

Saturated fat: 15%
Monounsaturated fat: 75%
Polyunsaturated fat: 10%

The more natural the fat, the better. Olive oil is by far the least processed of the oils we use and has a very high percentage of heart-healthy monounsaturated fat.

RICE BRAN OIL

Saturated fat: 25%
Monounsaturated fat: 38%
Polyunsaturated fat: 37%

Rice bran oil is a mild-flavoured oil with a high smoke point. It can therefore be used when high temperatures are needed, which make olive oil and butter unsuitable.

This oil has a much higher percentage of polyunsaturated fat than olive oil. Rice bran oil has some unique features, which balance the omega-6 content. Rice bran oil is rich in vitamin E and antioxidants, both of which have an anti-inflammatory effect and can help to lower levels of bad cholesterol.

RAPESEED OIL

Saturated fat: 7%
Monounsaturated fat: 61%
Polyunsaturated fat: 32%

Rapeseed oil, also known as canola oil, is another useful oil for cooking. It has a mild, earthy flavour and can be heated to high temperatures. It is a home-grown British oil that needs minimal processing to produce. Although a vegetable oil containing polyunsaturates, a high proportion of the polyunsaturates (33%) are omega-3s, which make it a healthy choice.

BUTTER

Saturated fat: 68%
Monounsaturated fat: 28%
Polyunsaturated fat: 4%

Cooking with butter is a great way to add flavour to meat or a sauce. It is high in filling saturated fat. As it contains some proteins and sugars it can burn easily so isn't suitable for frying.

Live bio cultures

Your gut is chock full of bacteria, good and bad. Live bio cultures are the good bacteria, otherwise known as probiotics, with which we can supplement our diet to help reverse the damage caused by years of eating a wheat- and sugar-rich diet. Live bio cultures can be found naturally in some foods, particularly yoghurt. But to really have an impact on our digestive systems, a probiotic supplement is the best way to ensure we have enough good bacteria to balance the gut effectively.

If your waist size varies during the day, certain foods make you gassy and uncomfortable or you suffer from any minor digestive complaints, you should consider a probiotic supplement in the form of a powder or tablet.

A typical probiotic supplement has the equivalent bacteria of at least four portions of natural yoghurt. Always read the packet and aim for the strongest concentration of bacteria. Supplements can range in strength from 1–450 billion bacteria.

The benefits of probiotics are hard to prove as you don't feel instantly better. It's more like planting a seed and waiting for it to grow. It is highly likely, however, that after a diet overloaded with bread and wheat products, your digestive tract is in need of some repair.

The most proven and the one now being prescribed by specialists for IBS and similar illnesses is a brand of probiotic called VSL3 (www.vsl3.co.uk). This brand contains the most strains of good bacteria and has 450 billion bacteria per sachet. But it is expensive and needs to be kept refrigerated. You may also find that such a high dosage is too strong for the current state of your gut, in which case you should start with a lower dose.

Other probiotics are cheaper and come in a simpler to take capsule form. Look for ones with at least four different strains of bacteria and a large quantity of bacteria, at least 10 billion per dose.

Whatever brand you choose, it's important that you take it for at least a month. It takes approximately three weeks for your gut to be recolonised with good bacteria. After that it's up to you. You may need to keep taking probiotics daily or you might find that you can cut back or switch to live yoghurt.

If you do stop taking them then it is useful to have some available to take if your stomach is under stress. Stomach stress triggers can include exhaustion, a tummy bug, food poisoning or a prolonged period of high wheat intake.

If you need to take antibiotics then these will kill off a lot of gut bacteria so it is wise to take a new course of probiotics after any antibiotics.

Finally, if you are planning on going abroad, particularly somewhere exotic, then it is worth boosting your probiotics before you go and during your travels. This will give you a stronger stomach for extra resistance, leaving you less open to stomach bugs and food poisoning.

To keep your gut in good health into the long term you should make sure you get a daily dose of probiotics in your food, together with a source of prebiotics. Prebiotics are bacteria nourishing foods that contain resistant starch (fibre). Good sources are green bananas, lentils, chickpeas and oats.

How they work

Processed food made from wheat and sugar contains ingredients that irritate the gut and cause bad bacteria to thrive. Eating too much processed food can inflame the gut lining and create small perforations in the cell walls. Partially digested food can slither through the cracks and cause inflammation and an unwanted immune response. By cutting out the wheat and sugar, the bad bacteria have less to feed on, and by taking extra probiotics you can rebuild a healthy digestive system and give the gut time to repair and strengthen.

How to take them

For the probiotics to be most effective it is best to take them on an empty stomach with lots of water. I find that the best time to take them is first thing in the morning at least half an hour before breakfast. Another good time would be just before bed, several hours after dinner.

Taking probiotics on an empty stomach helps the bacteria get past the acids in the stomach intact, allowing the majority of bacteria to reach the neutral intestines where they can grow and flourish.

What to expect

Most people don't experience any side effects when taking probiotics. It is, however, relatively common to experience bloating and gut discomfort in the first few days of taking them. This is due to the good bacteria trying to establish themselves in the gut. The symptoms should disappear in 3–7 days.

If you think that you are intolerant to foods such as milk, tomatoes or beans then probiotics may help. Remove the problematic food entirely from your diet when you start to take the probiotics. Let the probiotics start to work and when you feel your digestion is in good balanced health, try reintroducing the food in small doses. You may always be slightly wary of this food but you won't need to avoid it entirely.

Foods that contain probiotics

YOGHURT

The obvious choice. Full-fat natural yoghurt is the richest food source of probiotics. It normally contains two strains, lactobacillus and bifidobacterium, both known to help regulate the digestive system. Look for organic or live yoghurts. Yoghurts with a longer shelf life may well have been pasteurised, which kills off the probiotics.

KEFIR

Kefir is a natural fermented milk drink, which is very rich in probiotics. It is becoming more popular in the UK and can be found in health food shops.

CHEESE

Most cheese in the UK is made from pasteurised milk where all the friendly bacteria have sadly been removed. Home-made or farm cheese may well be unpasteurised. Look at the label as the manufacturer has a commitment to label the cheese as unpasteurised cheese will be unsuitable for pregnant women.

Unpasteurised hard cheeses can be a good source of probiotics. Cheddar, Gouda, feta and Parmesan, if unpasteurised, will all contain probiotics.

TAMARI SAUCE

Tamari is a Japanese wheat-free soy sauce. It is made from cultured soy beans and is a good probiotic source. Available from supermarkets, I now use this whenever a recipe calls for soy sauce.

PROBIOTICS IN COOKING

Heating probiotics over 40°C kills all the bacteria. This means that cooking with any probiotic foodstuffs will negate any gut health benefits. Yoghurt should be eaten chilled but can be stirred in to a dish after removing from the heat, which will preserve a proportion of the good bacteria. Tamari can be used to make a dip or a dressing for your food, which is added after cooking.

Living, shopping, planning

New essentials shopping list

On the following page is a basic shopping list of useful foods for your beautifully balanced wheat-free diet. If you choose to follow the meal planners you'll want to use this list as the bedrock of your diet, and then supplement with the extra list at the end of each weekly plan.

Fruit and veg
Apples
Blueberries
Strawberries
Lemons
Limes
Kiwis
Satsumas
Spring onions
Tomatoes
Cherry tomatoes
Cucumber
Salad leaves
Onion
Garlic
Ginger
Fresh chillies
Mushrooms
Courgettes
Red and green peppers
New potatoes
Butternut squash

Meat and fish
Chicken breast fillets
Salmon fillets
Lean minced beef
Streaky bacon or
pancetta
Cooked and peeled
king prawns
Ham
Chorizo

Store cupboard
Olive oil
Extra-virgin olive oil
Rice bran oil
Rapeseed oil
Balsamic vinegar
Basmati rice
Steamed brown rice
pouches
Oatcakes
Tomato purée
Garlic purée
Cornflour
Tamari soy sauce
Nam pla fish sauce
Tinned chopped
tomatoes
Coconut milk
Pine nuts
Cashews
Sunflower seeds
Ready-to-eat chickpeas
Ready-to-eat kidney
beans
Ready-to-eat haricot
beans
Paprika
Smoked paprika
Chilli flakes
Mild chilli powder
Ground cumin
Cumin seeds
Bay leaves
Olives
Piquante (Peppadew)
peppers
Roasted red peppers
Jalapeño peppers
Low-sugar jam
Clear honey

Baking
Ground almonds
Baking powder
Truvia® (natural stevia
sweetener)
Desiccated coconut
Dark chocolate
(70% cocoa solids)
Jumbo oats
Porridge oats
Cocoa powder
Vanilla bean paste

Dairy and chilled
Butter
Natural yoghurt
Greek yoghurt
Large free-range eggs
Full-fat milk
Cheddar
Feta
Parmesan
Halloumi

Frozen
Frozen peas
Frozen mixed berries

Baking essentials

Cakes and biscuits are a bit different without wheat flour. You'll find that they are denser and moist with a more crumbly texture. You'll also find them surprisingly filling and, because they won't give you a sugar high, you'll stay fuller for longer.

The ingredients you need can vary greatly from what you might expect. This is because the staple ingredients of all baking are wheat flour and sugar. You will discover new baking friends, some of which you won't even have heard of yet.

The biggest change to think about is to start using low-carbohydrate flours, namely almond flour and coconut flour. Other gluten-free flours such as rice flour are not recommended as they are an easy source of carbohydrate for the body so will raise blood sugar levels. If you stick to low-carb flours you can eat cakes guilt-free. These flours are becoming more readily available and can now be found in some supermarkets as well as online. Although they are relatively expensive, you use less of them than regular flours and they are well worth the investment. A new ingredient that is also important in wheat-free baking is xanthan gum. This

	Availability	Where to buy?
Coconut flour	Medium	Large supermarkets and health food shops
Almond flour	Low	A growing range of supermarkets. Currently Waitrose and Tesco.
Xanthan gum	Medium	Large supermarkets and health food shops
Oat bran	High	Most supermarkets

helps improve the crumb structure and reduce crumbling. It is now available in big supermarkets and health food shops.

Baking is doubly tricky as you need to replace both the flour and sugar in the recipe without compromising on taste or flavour. I use a natural sugar substitute in combination with sweet flavours such as fruit (fresh or dried), vanilla or even a little bit of honey. The recipes are never overly sweet because you'll find your need for sweetness reduces as your taste buds adjust to the new diet. My favourite option is Truvia® as it is a non-chemical sweetener derived from the stevia leaf. Sometimes I use 100% Truvia® but often I blend it with other sugars such as honey or brown sugar to bring a natural, balanced flavour without elevating sugar levels.

I also use vanilla bean paste in a lot of recipes. Vanilla bean paste is thicker than vanilla extract and contains vanilla bean seeds as well as a little sugar. It adds a gourmet taste and appearance to recipes.

Suppliers

The Asian Cookshop
Stocks a huge range of Asian foods, including shirataki noodles at a reasonable price.

Mexgrocer
Sells excellent 100% corn tortillas and masa harina corn flour

Sukrin
Sukrin sells almond and coconut flours – their products can be found in Tesco and Waitrose as well as online.

Your lifestyle, your diet

A little bit of planning will help make your diet so much easier. In the first week, when your body is still adapting to eating wheat-free, you may still experience cravings and be tempted to overeat. A 'no tolerance' approach during the first week will yield really good results. By week two, you'll be settling in to wheat-free eating and by week three and beyond you should find you no longer crave bread or wheat products.

If you work 9–5

- If you don't have time for a sit-down breakfast in the morning, make a wheat-free muffin or flapjack to munch on the way to work. Skipping breakfast will leave you more likely to overeat later in the day.
- Preparation is the key for lunch. Make a salad or microwave meal and take it with you. Don't rely on your local sandwich shop to provide you with something wheat-free.
- Tell your work colleagues that you are now eating gluten-free. That should stop them offering you cakes and treats from the snack table.
- Remember to avoid beer or lager if you go out for drinks after work. Wine or spirits are allowed.
- Stick to quick and easy dinners during the week but cook yourself a few treats at the weekend.

If you are single

- Don't be tempted by a take-away, it's so easy to overeat.
- If your cupboards are bare, an omelette makes a filling dinner.
- If you're out on a date, just decline the bread roll and choose good carbs for your main course.
- It's important not to skip meals, even if you don't feel particularly hungry.
- When cooking for friends a curry or moussaka makes a good dinner party dish. Wow your friends with a wheat-free dessert like Chocolate Hazelnut Torte (page 234). They'll be seriously impressed.

If you are a full-time mum

- If breakfast time is mayhem, you could have your breakfast after the kids have gone to school or playgroup. An omelette, a coffee and a sit down. Perfect.
- Find wheat-free alternatives to your family's favourite meals. A chilli makes a tasty change from spaghetti bolognaise. Try something new like fajitas, you may be pleasantly surprised.
- Be firm and never allow yourself to eat your children's crusts or leftovers.
- All children love yoghurts, so you can all have a healthy pudding together.
- Buy individual packs of biscuits or treats for your children

instead of a family size pack. An open packet of biscuits will always be a temptation.

If you are dieting as a couple

- Clear the cupboards of all biscuits and wheat-based treats. Remove beer from the house.
- Make a plan together and agree who is going to cook what.
- Going out for a nice meal is perfectly allowed. Just avoid pizza and pasta restaurants as they will offer you limited choices.
- A little bit of competitive spirit should spur you both on and make you less likely to cheat.

If you're a vegetarian

- Eat chickpeas, pulses and beans to boost your protein levels.
- Eggs and cheese are your friends. Remember you are allowed more fat now that you are curbing the carbs.
- If you are eating rice, add as many different vegetables as you can.
- Experiment with spicy options. Vegetable curries are fabulous. Try Fresh Saag Paneer (page 162) for a filling and quick veggie curry.
- Snacking on a variety of nuts will keep you full and provide extra protein.

Tips for eating out

Snacking on the go

When you are dashing about and need a quick pick-me-up, what should you reach for? The shelves are stacked full of wheat-filled junk food and it can feel like you've got no escape. But there are a few suitable snacks available at even the most disreputable establishments.

PEANUTS

Plain roasted and salted peanuts make a hugely satisfying snack. Available just about anywhere they are stock full of protein, fat and good carbs. A small snack pack can give you enough energy to last for up to 4 hours.

FLAPJACK

A flapjack is not 100% healthy as the sugar content will inevitably be high. But the oats will be filling and a flapjack is normally wheat-free. Check the ingredients for hidden wheat (it gets everywhere) and look for one that is natural, with the least number of ingredients as possible.

CADBURY'S FRUIT & NUT

For emergency use only! Wheat-free but stacked with sugar. The nuts add a little bit of extra protein.

Lunchtime eating

Your 'big 4' lunchtime choices are salad, soup, microwave hotpot and sushi.

All the major city chains such as Marks & Spencer, Pret a Manger, Costa and beyond offer a huge range of lunchtime options. The majority of their choices are sandwiches and wraps, but they all have a limited range of suitable alternatives.

A salad is perhaps the most obvious choice. Choose a salad that contains plenty of protein and/or complex carbohydrates such as beans or lentils. Ignore the calorie content on the pack and choose the most appetising and filling option.

If you have access to a microwave then soup is also a good option. Again choose the most appealing soups, preferably with lots of vegetables and beans. Some soups contain pasta so will need to be avoided. Always check the packaging for hidden wheat. Choose soups from the refrigerated aisle rather than a tin, as fresh soups contain more nutrients and less salt.

For vegetarians, the fresh meals in a pot from the chilled aisle in the supermarket are a healthy and filling option – as well as being quick and easy to heat in the microwave. They use flavours from around the world to make filling and versatile meals. Most, but not all, are wheat-free, so check the packet.

Sushi can be bought pre-packaged from the bigger chains. Sushi is often more expensive than other options but is filling and tasty. Be careful as some of the sauces contain gluten, although this should be clearly indicated on the pack.

Remember that as well as your main meal, there will be quite a lot of suitable snacks to accompany your lunch. Add a pack of nuts or peanuts if you are particularly hungry. For dessert, yoghurt options abound, as do pre-chopped fresh fruit. Most shops now also sell the tiny bars of dark chocolate, which make a great accompaniment to a cup of tea.

Choosing a restaurant

Eating out while avoiding wheat needn't be a chore. In fact, restaurant food can often be wheat-free as long as you skip the bread and pasta. If it's the kind of restaurant where the food is cooked fresh from scratch then there is unlikely to be added wheat in your meal. However, if you choose a fast food restaurant then quite a lot of the food will be prepared in advance and stored frozen, which inevitably means more ingredients and an increased risk of wheat. On the plus side, in a fast food or large restaurant chain, you will often see 'gluten free' marked on the menu besides certain dishes. This will guarantee that no wheat has been added to the dish.

It will depend on your level of sensitivity to wheat and gluten whether you specifically ask the waiter to check whether a dish is gluten-free. Don't feel embarrassed to do this, most staff will have been asked this many times before and will be able to check quite easily.

Finally, your enjoyment of the meal and the number of choices you are offered will depend on the style of food that they serve.

Top 5 restaurants for wheat-free	Top 5 restaurants to avoid for wheat-free
Traditional English or French restaurants Curry houses Japanese restaurants and sushi bars Upmarket burger bars (avoid the bun) Spicy chicken restaurants	Italian, pizza or pasta restaurants Fast food burger chains Fried chicken shops Fish and chips Bakeries

Complete 4-week plan

Use this detailed guide to organise your food choices for the week. This guide is intended to be as practical as possible, with quick weekday dinner choices and more complex meals and baking at the weekend. If a dish makes several portions then where possible you'll be able to keep leftovers and have them the next day. When a recipe contains meat or fish, then a vegetarian option will always be offered.

As you become more confident with wheat-free eating, feel free to replace a meal with a similar dish. I have tried to accommodate a really good balance of fat, protein and good carbs, as well as plenty of fruit and vegetables. There's also a few extra snacks and treats in weeks one and two. This will help you stick to the diet as your body adapts to the wheat-free lifestyle. By week three, you should find your need for extra snacks and treats will have diminished.

The majority of ingredients needed for the week are incorporated into the New Essentials Shopping List (page 67). Extra ingredients needed for each week are listed after each weekly meal plan.

Week 1

	Breakfast	Lunch	Dinner	Other
Mon	Omelette and cherry tomatoes	Lentil and Feta Salad (page 129)	Sweet and Sour Chicken with rice (page 174) or Veggie Chilli (page 176)	Choice of (max 3 per day)
Tues	Microwave Porridge (page 94)	Chorizo and Bean Stew (page 118) or Veggie Chilli (page 176)	Mediterranean Lamb Stew (page 149) or Moroccan Chickpea Stew (page 165)	· Chilli Spiced Nuts (page 108) · Natural yoghurt with 1 tsp honey
Wed	Omelette & ham	Mediterranean Lamb Stew (page 149) or Moroccan Chickpea Stew (page 165)	Courgette Spaghetti (page 135) with Hot Chilli Prawns (page 139) or with Easy Tomato Sauce (page 171)	· Fresh fruit – apple, kiwi, satsuma, blueberries or strawberries
Thurs	Bircher Muesli (page 96)	Greek Salad Plate (page 122)	Parmesan Chicken (page 142) with salad & new potatoes or Mushroom Stroganoff (page 143)	· 3 squares dark chocolate · Fruit and Nut Brownies (page 227)
Fri	Bircher Muesli (page 96)	Toasted Cumin Halloumi (page 123)	Salmon with Cajun Spice Rub (page 202) with new potatoes and broccoli or Courgette Spaghetti (page 135) with Sun-dried Tomato and Cashew Nut (page 140)	· Small glass red wine
Sat	Spanish Vegetable Tortilla (page 92)	Toasted Cumin Halloumi (page 123)	Roasted Red Pepper and Feta Tart (page 151)	
Sun	Continental Plate (page 97)	Roasted Red Pepper and Feta Tart (page 151)	Hot Steak Fajitas (page 144) or Thai Vegetable Curry (page 160)	

Week 1 shopping list

This is what you need in addition to the New Essentials Shopping List to follow the week 1 plan. Ingredients marked (V) are only needed if you are taking the vegetarian option.

Fruit and veg
Oranges
Little gem lettuce
Rocket leaves
Broccoli
Aubergine (V)
Flat-leaf parsley (V)
Red onion
Fresh basil
Babycorn
Mange tout

Meat and fish
Trimmed rump steak
Diced lamb
Fresh chicken stock

Dairy and chilled
Gouda cheese
Eggs (large)

Baking
Raisins
Dark brown sugar
Coconut flour
Xanthan gum
Caster sugar

Store cupboard
Elderflower cordial
Dried cranberries
Cinnamon
Cayenne pepper
Dried thyme
Dried oregano
Mixed nuts
Walnuts
Dried porcini mushrooms (V)
Dijon mustard (V)
English mustard
Walnut oil
Ready-to-eat puy lentils
Sun-dried tomatoes in oil
Lemongrass paste (V)
Red wine vinegar
White wine vinegar
Sherry
Ready-to-eat mixed beans
Red lentils (V)
Gram (chickpea) flour
Corn tortilla wraps

Week 2

	Breakfast	Lunch	Dinner	Other
Mon	Spanish Vegetable Tortilla (page 92)	Smoked Salmon & Cream Cheese Oatcakes (page 130) or roasted pepper and cream cheese on oatcakes	Indian Red Rice (page 193), grilled chicken and Chilli Lime Dip (page 200) or Indian Red Rice (page 193) with mushrooms and Chilli Lime Dip (page 200)	Choice of (max 3 per day) · Spicy Chickpeas (page 107)
Tues	Spanish Vegetable Tortilla (page 92)	Prawn and Avocado Salad (page 140) or Lentil and Feta Salad (page 129)	Turkish Kofta Kebabs (page 161) with Roasted Butternut Squash (page 197) or Mushroom Stroganoff (page 143) with Roasted Butternut Squash (page 197)	· Natural yoghurt with 1 tsp honey · Fresh fruit – apple, kiwi, satsuma, blueberries or strawberries
Wed	Scrambled egg with tomatoes and cheese	Paneer Curry Pot (page 124)	Courgette Spaghetti (page 135) with Monkfish and Chorizo (page 137) or Sun-dried Tomato and Cashew Nut (page 140)	· 3 squares dark chocolate
Thurs	Everyday Oats (page 96)	Paneer Curry Pot (page 124)	Spanish Baked Prawns (page 128) or Egg Florentine (page 145) with Three Pepper Pilau Rice (page 196)	· Coconut Crumbles (page 225)
Fri	Omelette and ham or Omelette and cheese	Mushroom and Bacon Rice (page 120) or Mushroom Rice	Piri Piri Chicken (page 164) with new potatoes and salad or Mexican Beans and Cheese (page 127)	· Small glass red wine
Sat	Continental Plate (page 97)	Japanese Noodle Salad (page 119) or Mexican Beans and Cheese (page 127)	Courgette Spaghetti (page 135) with Classic Bolognaise (page 183) or Lentil and Mushroom Bolognaise (page 155)	
Sun	Fruity Bran Loaf (page 93)	Baked Leek and Blue Cheese Frittata (page 131)	Lasagne with Courgette Pasta (page 184) or Lentil and Mushroom Bolognaise (page 155)	

Week 2 shopping list

This is what you need in addition to the New Essentials Shopping List to follow the week 2 plan. Ingredients marked (V) are only needed if you are taking the vegetarian option.

Fruit and veg	Store cupboard
Avocado	Gluten-free granola
Radishes	Ready-to-eat puy lentils
Iceberg lettuce	Tinned chickpeas
Leeks	Walnut oil (V)
Carrot (V)	English mustard (V)
Pak choi	Dijon mustard (V)
Rocket leaves (V)	Walnuts
Cabbage or spring greens	Dried puy lentils
Fresh mint	Shirataki noodles
Flat-leaf parsley	French mayonnaise
Bird's eye chillies	Porcini mushrooms (V)
	Sherry (V)
Meat and fish	Noilly Prat
Minced lamb	Vegetable stock (V)
Smoked salmon	Sun-dried tomatoes in oil (V)
Monkfish	Red wine vinegar
	White wine vinegar
Dairy and chilled	Black rice vinegar
Cream cheese	Tabasco
Paneer	Passata
Dolcelatte	Pesto
Eggs (large)	Worcestershire sauce
	Mushroom ketchup
Baking	Red wine
Oat bran	Cinnamon sticks
Sultanas	Cloves
Dried apricots	Turmeric
Dates	Cayenne pepper
Coconut flour	Chinese five-spice
Xanthan gum	Dried oregano
Brown sugar	Dried mixed herbs
	Dill
	Ground coriander
	Cinnamon

Week 3

	Breakfast	Lunch	Dinner	Other
Mon	Fruity Bran Loaf (page 93)	Egg Florentine (page 145)	Fresh Saag Paneer (page 162)	Choice of (max 2 per day)
Tues	Omelette and ham or Omelette and cheese	Oatcakes with Smoked Salmon and Cream Cheese (page 130) or Oatcakes with cream cheese and roasted peppers	Sesame Chicken Noodles (page 150) or Mushroom Stroganoff (page 143)	· Cinnamon Roasted Cashews (page 106) · Natural yoghurt with 1 tsp honey
Wed	Everyday Oats (page 96)	Greek Salad Plate (page 122)	Courgette Spaghetti (page 135) with Creamy Spicy Sausage (page 138) or Sun-dried Tomato and Cashew Nut (page 140)	· Fresh fruit – apple, kiwi, satsuma, blueberries or strawberries
Thurs	Scrambled eggs with tomatoes and cheese	Sticky Coconut Rice (page 195)	Chicken Casserole (page 178) with new potatoes and mangetout or Vegetarian Chilli (page 176) with rice	· 3 squares dark chocolate · Small glass red wine
Fri	Easy Microwave Porridge (page 94)	Chicken Casserole (page 178) or Vegetarian Chilli (page 176)	Hot Steak Fajitas (page 144) or Toasted Cumin Halloumi (page 123)	You can also add a pudding of your choice at the weekend
Sat	Smoked salmon and scrambled eggs or Omelette and cheese	Spanish Baked Prawns (page 128) or Toasted Cumin Halloumi (page 123)	Moussaka (page 169) and salad or Lentil and Mushroom Bolognaise (page 155)	
Sun	Choc Chip Banana Muffin (page 98)	Oriental Salmon Fishcakes (page 167) or Courgette Spaghetti (page 135) with Easy Tomato Sauce (page 171)	Orange and Lemon Chicken (page 158) with new potatoes and broccoli or Lentil and Mushroom Bolognaise (page 155)	

Week 3 shopping list

This is what you need in addition to the New Essentials Shopping List to follow the week 3 plan. Ingredients marked (V) are only needed if you are taking the vegetarian option.

Fruit and veg
Oranges
Little gem lettuce
Red onion
Fresh coriander
Basil (V)
Aubergines
Pak choi
Baby spinach
Carrots
Parsnips
Leeks
Broccoli
Mangetout

Meat and fish
Rump steak
Minced lamb
Fresh chicken stock
Streaky bacon
Smoked salmon
Cooked chicken
Smoked pork sausage

Dairy and chilled
Cream cheese
Paneer
Double cream
Eggs (large)

Frozen
Frozen Mediterranean vegetables

Store cupboard
Wheat-free granola
Corn tortilla wraps
Mayonnaise
White wine vinegar
Brown or green lentils (V)
Porcini mushrooms (V)
Dijon mustard
Wholegrain mustard
Walnut oil
Sesame oil
Gram (chickpea) flour
Passata
Tabasco
Sun-dried tomatoes in oil (V)
Vegetable stock cubes (V)
Sesame seeds
Cayenne pepper
Ground nutmeg
Ground cloves
Dill
Ground coriander
Dried thyme
Dried oregano
Turmeric
Cinnamon
Sherry (V)
White wine
Red wine (V)

Baking
Brown sugar

Week 4

	Breakfast	Lunch	Dinner	Other
Mon	Choc Chip Banana Muffin (page 98)	Puy Lentil and Feta Salad (page 129)	Sausage Hotpot (page 175) or Thai Vegetable Curry (page 160)	Choice of (max 2 per day) · Wasabi peas (page 111) · Natural yoghurt with 1 tsp honey · Fresh fruit – apple, kiwi, satsuma, blueberries or strawberries · 3 squares dark chocolate · Small glass red wine You can also add a pudding of your choice at the weekend
Tues	Choc Chip Banana Muffin (page 98)	Sausage Hotpot (page 175) or Thai Vegetable Curry (page 160)	Tabbouleh Parsley Salad (page 187) and Falafel Burgers (page 188)	
Wed	Bircher Muesli (page 96)	Tabbouleh Parsley Salad (page 187) and Falafel Burgers (page 188)	Salmon with Cajun Spice Rub (page 202) with new potatoes and broccoli or Sticky Coconut Rice (page 195)	
Thurs	Bircher Muesli (page 96)	Mexican Beans and Cheese (page 127)	Smoky Pork 'Chilli' (page 186) with rice or Vegetarian Chilli (page 176) with rice	
Fri	Easy Microwave Porridge (page 94)	Smoky Pork 'Chilli' (page 186) with rice or Vegetarian Chilli (page 176) with rice	Chicken Caesar Salad (page 132) or Courgette Spaghetti (page 135) with Sun-dried Tomato and Cashew Nut (page 140)	
Sat	Spanish Vegetable Tortilla (page 92)	Chorizo and Bean Stew (page 118) or Greek Salad Plate (page 122)	Beef Curry (page 156) with Big Indian Green Rice (page 192) or Red Pepper and Feta Tart (page 151)	
Sun	Spanish Vegetable Tortilla (page 92)	Courgette Spaghetti (page 135) and Hot Chilli Prawns (page 139) or Red Pepper and Feta Tart (page 151)	Moroccan Chickpea Stew (page 165)	

Week 4 shopping list

This is what you need in addition to the New Essentials Shopping List to follow the week 4 plan. Ingredients marked (V) are only needed if you are taking the vegetarian option.

Fruit and veg	Store cupboard
Rocket leaves	Elderflower cordial
Iceberg lettuce	Dried cranberries
Cos lettuce	Walnut oil
Cooked beetroot	English mustard
Aubergine	French mayonnaise
Babycorn (V)	White wine vinegar
Mangetout (V)	Ready-to-eat puy lentils
Broccoli	Ready-to-eat mixed beans
Pak choi (V)	Worcestershire sauce
Basil	Butterbeans
Flat-leaf parsley	Quinoa
Fresh Coriander	Almond butter
	Dried red lentils
Meat and fish	Capers
Gluten-free sausages	Sun-dried tomatoes in oil (V)
Fresh chicken stock	Black treacle
Lean pork mince	Harissa paste
Stewing beef steak	Gram (chickpea) flour
Cooked chicken breast	Bicarbonate of soda (V)
	Walnuts
Dairy and chilled	Dried oregano
Eggs (large)	Dried thyme
	Lemongrass paste (V)
	Ground cinnamon
	Ground coriander
	Ground nutmeg
	Ground cloves
	Ground ginger
	Cayenne pepper
	Caraway seeds
	Fennel seeds
	Cardamom pods
	Garam masala

RECIPE KEY

Preparation time:

Cooling Time:

Freezing time:

Resting time:

Cooking time:

    Oven

    Hob

    Microwave

Calories per serving: **174** calories

Recipes

5

Breakfast Basics

Breakfast is the most important meal of the day. You've probably heard that a lot but what you eat at breakfast controls what you eat during the day. Ideally it should be protein-rich, with only the best, most filling carbohydrates getting a look in. It's often a good time to get your daily dose of probiotics with the addition of some lovely natural yoghurt. Think oats, eggs and dairy as the key breakfast options.

A good breakfast will keep you generously full until lunchtime. This is important because if you are starving by lunch, there's a good chance you'll over-eat then and into the afternoon. You should also consider whether you will be exercising during the day. If you are going to be doing physical exercise, then I think having some good protein such as eggs is really important as that will give you the power to do a good workout.

My favourite simple start to the day is a 2-egg omelette (I'd recommend three eggs for a man), with a few halved cherry tomatoes on the side and an accompanying cup of good white coffee. I find that an omelette is the quickest and easiest egg dish to make in the morning. Heat a drizzle of rice bran oil in a heavy-based frying pan for a minute or two, before adding well-beaten eggs. Let the eggs cook a little before using a plastic spatula to pick up the sides of the omelette and letting the still runny centre go towards the edges. When just cooked (still a little wobbly in the middle), season with salt and pepper and fold in half before tipping onto a plate. It's ready in 2 minutes flat and I usually just wipe round the pan with some kitchen paper rather than washing it with soapy water; this will mean it's well-oiled for the next day.

If this is still too slow for you and you need a 'grab it and go' type breakfast, then try Bircher Muesli (page 96) or Everyday Oats (page 96). These combine good-quality carbohydrates, a little protein and lovely live cultures.

Perfect pecan granola

I love this granola. I've tried many different recipes over the years and this is the winner for me. Serve with milk, yoghurt or have a sneaky handful as a sweet snack.

SERVES 8   5 mins   20 mins

174 calories

200g jumbo oats
50g pecans, roughly chopped
30g butter
3 tbsp rice bran oil
2 tbsp (30g) soft dark brown sugar
1 tbsp (20g) maple syrup

Healthy fats	✓
Good carbs	✓
Low sugar	✓

Preheat the oven to 160°C/140°C fan/325°F/gas mark 3 and line a baking tray with baking parchment. Mix the oats and pecans together in a large bowl.

Heat the butter, oil, sugar and syrup together in a small pan and stir until completely combined and the sugar has dissolved. Pour over the oats and pecans and stir thoroughly.

Spread the granola out on the lined baking tray in a thin layer. Clumps and gaps are fine here, just make sure it's reasonably well spread out. Bake in the oven for 20 minutes, stirring halfway through to break up any big bits and make sure it's not stuck to the tray.

Leave to cool completely on the tray before transferring to an airtight container. The granola will keep for up to 10 days.

Spanish vegetable tortilla

If you think eggs are worth a try for breakfast but don't want to be cooking and prepping first thing in the morning, a tortilla is a very good bet. The eggs are cooked slowly with vegetables and then left to cool before cutting into slices. Stick it in the fridge overnight and it will be ready and waiting for: a filling and perfectly balanced breakfast. Just add coffee!

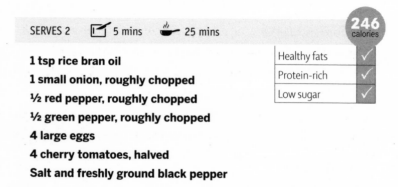

SERVES 2   5 mins   25 mins

246 calories

1 tsp rice bran oil

1 small onion, roughly chopped

½ red pepper, roughly chopped

½ green pepper, roughly chopped

4 large eggs

4 cherry tomatoes, halved

Salt and freshly ground black pepper

Healthy fats	✓
Protein-rich	✓
Low sugar	✓

Heat the oil in a small, lidded frying pan over a medium/high heat. Toss in the onion and peppers and season generously with salt and pepper. Cook over a medium heat until sizzling and then stir, reduce the heat to low and place the lid (or a suitably sized plate) on top. Cook for a further 10 minutes until soft. Remove the vegetables from the pan and set aside.

Whisk the eggs together in a bowl or jug and pour into the frying pan. After a couple of minutes, use a plastic spatula or fish slice to lift up the cooked edge of the eggs and allow the uncooked egg to run underneath. Continue to do this all round the pan. Then return the cooked vegetables to the pan, add the tomatoes and put the lid on. Cook for around 10 minutes, or until the eggs in the centre are just firm.

Flip the tortilla over on to a plate and leave to cool completely before cutting into quarters or wedges. The tortilla will keep for 48 hours in the fridge.

Fruity bran loaf

This fibre-rich loaf has no added sugar or sweetener but watch out: with all the dried fruit it contains, this loaf is relatively high in quick-release carbohydrates. Stick to one slice, either on its own or spread with a little butter or cream cheese.

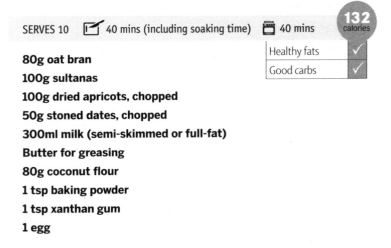

SERVES 10   40 mins (including soaking time)   40 mins   **132** calories

| Healthy fats | ✓ |
| Good carbs | ✓ |

80g oat bran
100g sultanas
100g dried apricots, chopped
50g stoned dates, chopped
300ml milk (semi-skimmed or full-fat)
Butter for greasing
80g coconut flour
1 tsp baking powder
1 tsp xanthan gum
1 egg

Place the oat bran and dried fruit in a bowl and pour over the milk. Stir and then leave to soak for at least 30 minutes.

Preheat the oven to 180°C/160°C fan/350°F/gas mark 4. Grease a small loaf tin and line the base with baking parchment.

In a large mixing bowl, combine the coconut flour, baking powder and xanthan gum.

Whisk the egg into the milk and fruit mixture and then add this to the flour; stir well. You are looking for a gloopy dough so if the mixture feels too firm, add about 3 tablespoons of water. Scoop the mixture into the prepared loaf tin and bake for 40 minutes until golden brown on the top.

Leave to cool completely before slicing. This loaf can be frozen as a whole or in individual slices.

Easy microwave porridge

This is my foolproof way to make great porridge. Delicious served plain or topped with fresh fruit, low-sugar jam or a home-made compote.

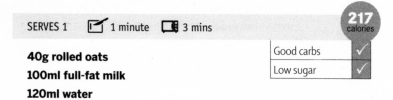

SERVES 1	1 minute	3 mins		**217** calories

40g rolled oats
100ml full-fat milk
120ml water

Good carbs	✓
Low sugar	✓

Simply combine the oats, milk and water in a high-sided microwave-safe bowl or jug.

Microwave on high power for 3 minutes. Stir thoroughly and add a little extra milk if necessary to gain the right consistency.

Red berry compote

A compote, especially when made with frozen fruits, is incredibly simple to make. The only addition is water so you can be absolutely sure that you're getting all of the goodness and nothing else. Red fruits such as strawberries, raspberries and cherries work particularly well.

If you prefer your compote a little sweeter, try adding a teaspoon of sugar or stevia at the end of the cooking time.

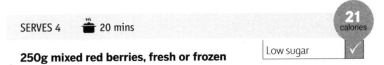

SERVES 4   20 mins   **21** calories

250g mixed red berries, fresh or frozen   Low sugar ✓

Place the fruits in a non-stick pan and cover generously with water.

Place the pan over a medium/high heat and bring to the boil. Reduce the heat so that the water is at a vigorous simmer and cook for about 20 minutes, topping up with more water if necessary.

When cooked the fruit should be starting to break up but not completely smooth. Leave to cool in the pan and then transfer to a glass dish. Cover and refrigerate. The compote will keep for up to 5 days.

Everyday oats

This is another oaty favourite of mine and can be ready on the table in 2 minutes flat. Make sure the granola is a gluten-free recipe or make your own.

SERVES 1   2 mins   **260** calories

30g jumbo oats
200ml milk
1 tbsp Greek yoghurt
10g granola

Good carbs	✓
Probiotics	✓
Low sugar	✓

Simply mix the oats, milk and yoghurt together in a bowl, sprinkle the granola over the top and enjoy.

Bircher muesli

This is one of my favourite breakfast dishes at the moment. Make it up in a few minutes, tip it back into the yoghurt pot and it's ready to serve up for breakfast for the next few days. Be sure to use a yoghurt with no added sugars or flavourings and check that it is not low fat.

SERVES 4   2 mins   **113** calories

500g natural yoghurt
2 tsp stevia
1 tsp elderflower cordial
10g dried cranberries
20g jumbo rolled oats

Good carbs	✓
Probiotics	✓
Low sugar	✓

Simply tip the yoghurt out into a bowl and stir through the stevia, elderflower cordial, cranberries and oats. If it's too thick, add a little water and stir again.

Serve immediately or scoop back into the yoghurt pot and chill overnight so the oats and yoghurt are soaked through and ready for tomorrow's breakfast.

Continental plate

Sometimes a good breakfast is all about presentation. This cold plate of meat and cheese is both filling and appetising. This is a great alternative to a greasy fry-up when you want to avoid carbs at breakfast.

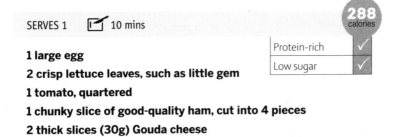

SERVES 1   10 mins   **288** calories

Protein-rich	✓
Low sugar	✓

1 large egg
2 crisp lettuce leaves, such as little gem
1 tomato, quartered
1 chunky slice of good-quality ham, cut into 4 pieces
2 thick slices (30g) Gouda cheese

First lightly boil your egg by placing it gently into a pan of simmering water. Cook for 7–9 minutes, depending on how you like it cooked. Remove from the pan with a slotted spoon and cool for a few minutes before peeling and cutting into quarters.

Arrange the lettuce and tomatoes over one side of the plate, with the ham and cheese arranged on the other side. Finally place the quartered egg in the centre.

Vanilla yoghurt

A fresh and simple way to start the day. Delicious on its own or served with a handful of fresh berries.

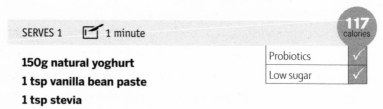

SERVES 1   1 minute   **117** calories

150g natural yoghurt
1 tsp vanilla bean paste
1 tsp stevia

| Probiotics | ✓ |
| Low sugar | ✓ |

Simply mix the ingredients together and serve.

Choc chip banana muffins

These are really good muffins. They are low in sugar and full of good stuff to help you start the day.

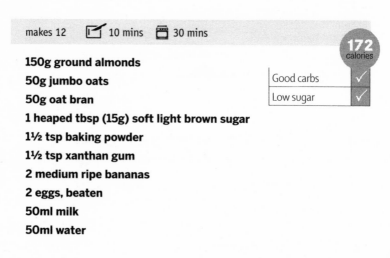

makes 12   10 mins   30 mins   **172** calories

150g ground almonds
50g jumbo oats
50g oat bran
1 heaped tbsp (15g) soft light brown sugar
1½ tsp baking powder
1½ tsp xanthan gum
2 medium ripe bananas
2 eggs, beaten
50ml milk
50ml water

| Good carbs | ✓ |
| Low sugar | ✓ |

50g dark chocolate chips
12 brown paper cases

Preheat the oven to 180°C/160°C fan/350°F/gas mark 4. Line a cupcake tin with 12 paper cases.

In a large bowl, thoroughly mix the ground almonds, oats, oat bran, brown sugar, baking powder and xanthan gum.

Mash the bananas to a pulp with the back of a fork in a separate bowl. Add the eggs, milk and water and stir to combine. Pour over the dry ingredients and stir to make a wet dough. Stir through the chocolate chips.

Spoon the dough into the prepared cases and bake in the oven for 30 minutes.

Remove from the oven and leave to rest in the tin for 5 minutes. When cool enough to handle, transfer to a cooling rack. Store in an airtight container for up to a week; alternatively these muffins can be frozen.

Home-made beans

These have no added sugar or sweeteners and are really quick to make. You won't want to go back to shop-bought beans after trying these ones. Serve with scrambled eggs and bacon.

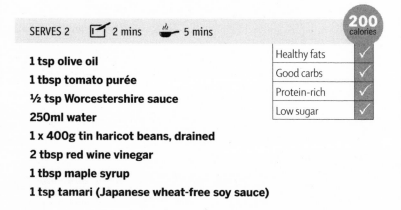

SERVES 2   2 mins   5 mins   **200** calories

Healthy fats	✓
Good carbs	✓
Protein-rich	✓
Low sugar	✓

1 tsp olive oil
1 tbsp tomato purée
½ tsp Worcestershire sauce
250ml water
1 x 400g tin haricot beans, drained
2 tbsp red wine vinegar
1 tbsp maple syrup
1 tsp tamari (Japanese wheat-free soy sauce)

Heat the oil in a pan over a low heat. Add the tomato purée and fry for a minute before adding the Worcestershire sauce, water and drained beans.

Increase the heat and bring to a simmer before adding the red wine vinegar, maple syrup and tamari. Cook gently over a low heat for 5 minutes.

Serve immediately or allow to cool and refrigerate (these beans only improve in flavour) for up to 2 days. Simply reheat gently before serving.

6

Simple Snacks

Japanese roasted edamame

Have you tried edamame beans in Japanese restaurants and wondered how to make them yourself? Or you may even have heard that they are Victoria Beckham's favourite food? Well here's the simple truth. Edamame are just baby soya beans and you can get them in any supermarket. What's more, they are incredibly simple to cook. Feel free to experiment with different flavours.

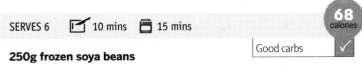

SERVES 6   10 mins   15 mins   **68** calories

Good carbs ✓

250g frozen soya beans
2 tsp sesame oil
½ tsp salt
½ tsp chilli flakes

Spread the soya beans out on kitchen paper to defrost. Pat dry with more kitchen paper before cooking as the beans need to be dry to stay crunchy.

Preheat the oven to 200°C/180°C fan/350°F/gas mark 4.

Mix the sesame oil, salt and chilli flakes in a bowl and add the soya beans. Toss through so each is thoroughly coated. Pour the soya beans on to a baking tray and shake to distribute evenly across the tray. Bake in the preheated oven for 12–15 minutes, turning them halfway through cooking. Leave to cool completely on the tray. These are best eaten the same day but can be kept in an airtight container for a day or two.

Crunchy kale 'seaweed'

Spring greens or cabbage also work well in this dish. It's really easy and the seaweed is very, very moreish.

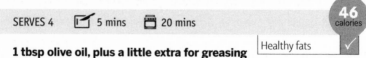

SERVES 4   5 mins   20 mins   **46** calories

Healthy fats ✓

1 tbsp olive oil, plus a little extra for greasing
150g curly kale, washed and dried well
1 tsp walnut oil
1 tsp Chinese five-spice powder
1 tbsp gluten-free soy sauce

Preheat the oven to 160°C/140°C fan/325°F/gas mark 3 and lightly grease two baking trays with a little olive oil.

Cut the kale leaves into thin strips, about ½ cm wide. Discard any discoloured leaf parts and all the tough stems.

Place the strips into a large bowl. Add the walnut oil, olive oil, five-spice powder and soy sauce. Toss thoroughly with your hands; it's really important to get all the strips coated.

Distribute the kale strips evenly over the two baking trays. Bake for around 20 minutes until the leaves are dry and crunchy. Serve hot or cold.

Parsnip crisps

Parsnips make a healthier alternative to potatoes and give these crisps a distinctive earthy flavour.

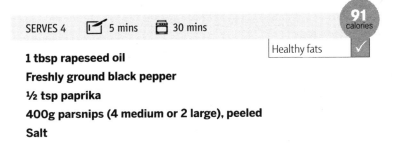

SERVES 4   5 mins   30 mins   **91** calories

| Healthy fats | ✓ |

1 tbsp rapeseed oil
Freshly ground black pepper
½ tsp paprika
400g parsnips (4 medium or 2 large), peeled
Salt

Preheat the oven to 160°C/140°C fan/325°F/gas mark 3.

Place the oil, pepper and paprika in a large bowl. Use a vegetable peeler to slice thin strips of parsnip into the bowl. Use your hands to toss the parsnip thoroughly in the oil.

Arrange the parsnip strips over two baking trays and then place in the preheated oven to cook for 25–30 minutes, turning them halfway through cooking. When cooked they will be golden and crisp.

Transfer to two large plates lined with kitchen paper and sprinkle liberally with salt.

Cinnamon roasted cashews

Cashews are a favourite snack of mine – they taste gorgeous simply sprinkled with a little salt. This recipe makes a more adventurous alternative; sweet and salty in equal measure. I've used a small quantity of brown sugar in this recipe. Alternatively you could replace this with an equivalent amount of stevia or artificial sweetener.

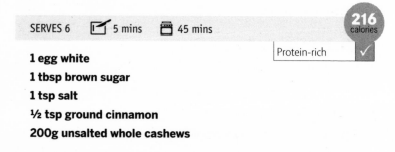

SERVES 6   5 mins   45 mins   **216** calories

Protein-rich ✓

1 egg white
1 tbsp brown sugar
1 tsp salt
½ tsp ground cinnamon
200g unsalted whole cashews

Preheat the oven to 140°C/120°C fan/275°F/gas mark 1 and line a baking tray with baking parchment.

Whisk the egg white until light and frothy and then mix in the sugar, salt and cinnamon. Add the cashews and stir until thoroughly coated. Spread evenly over the baking tray.

Bake in the oven for 45 minutes, stirring every 15 minutes until they are golden brown. Remove from the oven and allow to cool completely on the tray. Store in an airtight container.

Spicy chickpeas

A really easy to throw together snack, these chickpeas are simply roasted in the oven with a few spices.

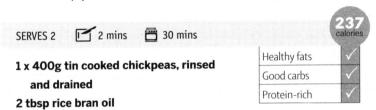

SERVES 2   2 mins   30 mins

237 calories

1 x 400g tin cooked chickpeas, rinsed and drained

2 tbsp rice bran oil

1 tsp salt

½ tsp hot chilli powder

1 tsp ground cumin

Healthy fats	✓
Good carbs	✓
Protein-rich	✓

Preheat the oven to 210°C/190°C fan/400°F/gas mark 6.

Pat dry the rinsed chickpeas with kitchen paper and pour into a bowl. Add the oil, salt, chilli powder and cumin and mix until well coated.

Spread the chickpeas in an even layer over a large baking tray and bake for approximately 30 minutes, until golden brown. Give them a gently shake every 10 minutes to make sure they bake evenly.

Leave to cool on the tray before eating or storing. The chickpeas will keep for 2–3 days in an airtight container.

Chilli spiced nuts

I make these amazing nuts often and store in a glass jar. Great for when you fancy a savoury snack or when you're feeling peckish at work. I've also proudly served them to friends and they disappeared incredibly quickly. Feel free to substitute with other types of nuts.

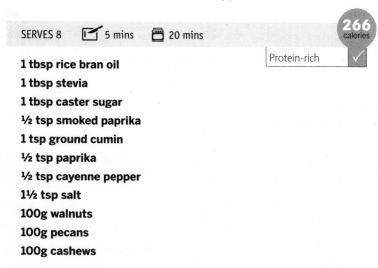

SERVES 8   5 mins   20 mins   **266** calories

Protein-rich ✓

1 tbsp rice bran oil
1 tbsp stevia
1 tbsp caster sugar
½ tsp smoked paprika
1 tsp ground cumin
½ tsp paprika
½ tsp cayenne pepper
1½ tsp salt
100g walnuts
100g pecans
100g cashews

Preheat the oven to 160°C/140°C fan/325°F/gas mark 3.

Combine the oil, stevia, sugar, spices and salt together in a small bowl and whisk together with a fork.

Combine the nuts in a bowl and pour over the flavoured oil; use your hands to mix thoroughly.

Put the nuts on a baking tray and bake for 15–20 minutes until fragrant and browned.

Cool completely on the tray and store in an airtight container until needed. These nuts will keep for about a week.

Corn tortillas

Corn tortillas are surprisingly easy to make, and are great for wraps or just for snacking. You will need a special flour called masa harina. This can be found in some specialist or health food shops or online; www.mexgrocer.co.uk is a good place to try.

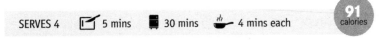

SERVES 4   5 mins   30 mins   4 mins each   **91** calories

100g masa harina
½ tsp salt
70ml boiling water
70ml tap water

Combine the masa harina and salt in a bowl. Measure out the boiling water and tap water together into a jug. Pour the water into the flour slowly, bringing the dough together with a spoon. When all the water has been added, knead lightly and bring together into a dough. Wrap in cling film and refrigerate for about 30 minutes.

Divide the dough into four equal pieces and roll each into a smooth ball. The easiest way to roll out the dough without it sticking is to cut a large freezer bag in half and place one ball between the two sheets of plastic. Roll out into a circle about 15cm in diameter and 2–3mm thick.

Heat a heavy-based frying pan over a high heat until very hot. Add the tortilla and cook undisturbed for 1–2 minutes, until the edges start to come away from the pan. Use a plastic spatula to turn the tortilla over and cook for a further minute.

Eat immediately or wrap in a damp tea towel and set aside while you make the rest of the tortillas. This will make the tortillas softer and more pliable.

Stuffed pickles

There are lots of strong flavours here, making this an awesome snack that it easy to put together. I use sweet piquante peppers (such as Peppadew) or red jalapeños.

makes 8 filled halves   5 mins

101 calories

Protein-rich ✓

4 pickled gherkins in sweet vinegar, drained
100g mild Cheddar, grated
3 tbsp mayonnaise
1½ tbsp pickled chilli peppers, drained and finely chopped

Cut the gherkins in half lengthways and use a teaspoon to scrape out the seeds down the centre of the pickle. Pat dry with kitchen paper.

In a small bowl, mix the cheese, mayonnaise and chopped chilli peppers. Use a knife to spread the mixture over each of the halved gherkins. Serve immediately.

Wasabi peas

Oh my word – these are soooo good! I use chickpeas for this recipe as I find they retain their bite really well when cooked.

SERVES 4   5 mins   40 mins   **118** calories

1x 400g tin chickpeas, rinsed and drained

1 tbsp olive oil

Sea salt

6 tsp wasabi powder

4 tsp water

1 tsp sesame oil

1 tbsp rice vinegar

1 tsp onion powder

Healthy fats	✓
Good carbs	✓
Protein-rich	✓

Preheat the oven to 220°C/200°C fan/425°F/gas mark 7.

Pat the chickpeas dry with kitchen paper and spread out on a baking tray. Drizzle over the olive oil and toss through until each chickpea is well coated. Sprinkle generously with sea salt and bake in the oven for 30 minutes.

Meanwhile prepare the wasabi sauce. Mix 4 teaspoons of the wasabi powder with 2 teaspoons of the water and leave for a few minutes for the flavour to develop. Then add the sesame oil, rice vinegar and half the onion powder, stir and leave to rest until the chickpeas have finished their first bake.

Remove the chickpeas from the oven and pour the wasabi sauce over. Toss the sauce through until the chickpeas are evenly coated. Return to the oven and bake for another 10 minutes until the peas are golden.

Make up a second batch of wasabi paste with the remaining 2 teaspoons of wasabi powder, 2 teaspoons of water and the rest of the onion powder. Stir through the cooked chickpeas and leave to cool completely on the baking tray.

Store in an airtight jar. These are great as a snack or as an alternative salad topping.

Parmesan oat crackers

These amazing savoury biscuits are delicious eaten on their own or with a chunk of your favourite cheese. Equally perfect as a late night snack or for dinner party entertaining.

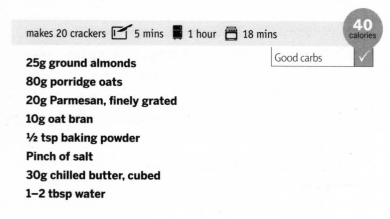

makes 20 crackers   5 mins   1 hour   18 mins   **40** calories

Good carbs ✓

25g ground almonds
80g porridge oats
20g Parmesan, finely grated
10g oat bran
½ tsp baking powder
Pinch of salt
30g chilled butter, cubed
1–2 tbsp water

In a large bowl, mix together the ground almonds, oats, Parmesan, oat bran, baking powder and salt. Add the cubed butter and rub in with your fingers until the mixture resembles breadcrumbs.

Start to bring the breadcrumbs together into a dough, adding a tablespoon of water to make a slightly moist but malleable dough.

Roll out into a thick sausage, the diameter of a £2 coin. Flatten the ends, wrap in cling film and chill thoroughly in the fridge for at least 1 hour or in the freezer for 15–20 minutes.

Preheat the oven to 190°C/170°C fan/375°F/gas mark 5.

Using your sharpest knife, cut the dough sausage into thin cylindrical slices, about 2–3mm thick. If you find that the dough collapses and falls apart as you cut it, it needs to be chilled some more. Lay out the slices on a baking tray and bake in the oven for 16–18 minutes until golden. Leave to cool completely on the baking tray before transferring to an airtight container.

Chocolate pecans

These are so easy to make, yet are a great healthy sweet snack. Don't rush melting the chocolate as it can turn white if cooled too quickly.

SERVES 4   5 mins

230 calories

Protein-rich ✓

100g whole pecans
40g dark chocolate (70% cocoa solids)
½ tsp stevia

Arrange the pecans on a tray covered with baking parchment. The pecans need to be in a flat single layer and very close together so you can barely see any paper underneath.

Chop up the chocolate into small pieces and place in a small microwaveable bowl. Heat on high in 10-second blasts, stirring carefully after each blast. When more than half of the chocolate has melted, remove from the microwave and keep stirring until it is completely smooth. Stir in the stevia.

As soon as the chocolate has totally melted, use a teaspoon to drizzle the chocolate over the pecans, making sure each pecan gets some chocolate. Leave to solidify on the tray and then transfer to an airtight container for storage. These will keep for up to 5 days, but I guarantee they won't last that long!

7

Lovely Lunches

Are you used to reaching for a quick sandwich for lunchtime refuelling? Now is the time to be a bit more adventurous. A little planning earlier in the day (or the evening before) pays dividends here. If you're finding it hard to turn away from your local sandwich shop, here are loads of options for quick and easy salads, soups and rice dishes. And if you want a hot meal there are plenty of options too, such as the delicious Paneer Curry Pot (page 124) or Toasted Cumin Halloumi with Butternut Squash (page 123).

Chorizo and bean stew

This recipe takes less than ten minutes to cook and is wonderfully filling. For the mixed beans, I prefer to use the kind that come vacuum-packed and ready to eat, although tinned beans work just as well; just rinse and drain well before using.

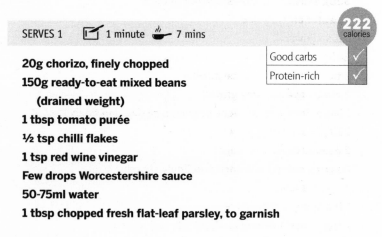

SERVES 1   1 minute   7 mins

222 calories

20g chorizo, finely chopped
150g ready-to-eat mixed beans
   (drained weight)
1 tbsp tomato purée
½ tsp chilli flakes
1 tsp red wine vinegar
Few drops Worcestershire sauce
50-75ml water
1 tbsp chopped fresh flat-leaf parsley, to garnish

Good carbs	✓
Protein-rich	✓

Place a small frying pan over a high heat until hot. Add the chopped chorizo and fry until turning brown on all sides, about 1–2 minutes.

Reduce the heat to low and then add in the beans, tomato purée, chilli flakes, vinegar, Worcestershire sauce and water. Stir well to combine. Allow the stew to start bubbling gently and then cook for another 5 minutes, stirring occasionally. Serve immediately, garnished with chopped parsley.

Japanese noodle salad

This is perhaps my favourite recipe using shirataki noodles. It's unusual, fresh and delicious.

SERVES 4 10 mins 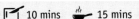 15 mins

Protein-rich ✓

300g shirataki noodles, soaked in warm water and drained

1 tbsp olive oil

200g minced beef

2 tsp Chinese five-spice powder

2 cloves garlic, finely grated

1 large thumb-sized piece of ginger, peeled and finely grated

250g cooked king prawns

2 heaped tsp brown sugar

6 spring onions, trimmed and finely sliced

Juice of 1 lime

1 tsp nam pla fish sauce

2 tsp tamari (Japanese wheat-free soy sauce)

1 red chilli, seeded and finely sliced

Handful of fresh coriander, chopped

2 fresh mint leaves, chopped

Freshly ground black pepper

In a wok or large frying pan, dry fry the noodles for 5–7 minutes until bone dry and cooked through. Set aside.

Heat the oil in the same pan over a medium heat and add the minced beef and five-spice powder. Fry until well browned. Add the garlic, ginger, prawns, brown sugar and spring onions. Cook for 3–4 minutes.

Place the cooled noodles in a large bowl with the lime juice, nam pla, tamari, red chilli, coriander, mint and black pepper. Stir through and divide between four plates. Serve the beef and prawn mixture over the noodles. Serve hot or cold.

Mushroom and bacon rice

This is an earthy wintry dish that is really filling and easy to make. It uses cooked brown rice and – I must confess – I often use the pre-steamed rice packs. Any green winter veg works well here, so feel free to experiment with whatever is in your fridge. Using ready-cooked rice means you can have this dish on the table in under 10 minutes.

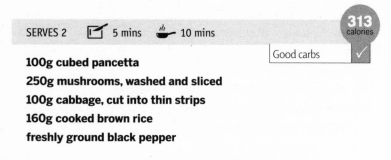

SERVES 2   5 mins   10 mins

313 calories

Good carbs ✓

100g cubed pancetta
250g mushrooms, washed and sliced
100g cabbage, cut into thin strips
160g cooked brown rice
freshly ground black pepper

Place a wide, lidded frying pan over a high heat and add the pancetta cubes. Fry until browned all over, about 4 minutes. Remove the pancetta from the pan using a slotted spoon and set aside.

Keeping the heat on high, toss the mushrooms into the pan and fry in the fat from the pancetta. Cook until browned and glistening, then remove and set aside.

Add the sliced cabbage to the pan, stir through and reduce the heat to low. Add a tablespoon of water and place the lid on

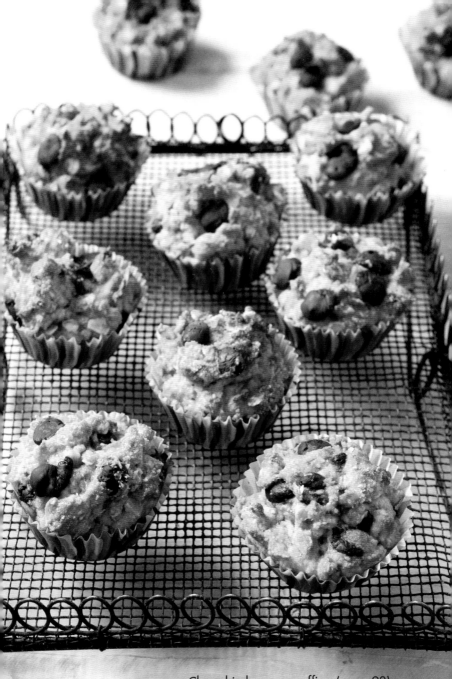

Choc chip banana muffins (page 98)

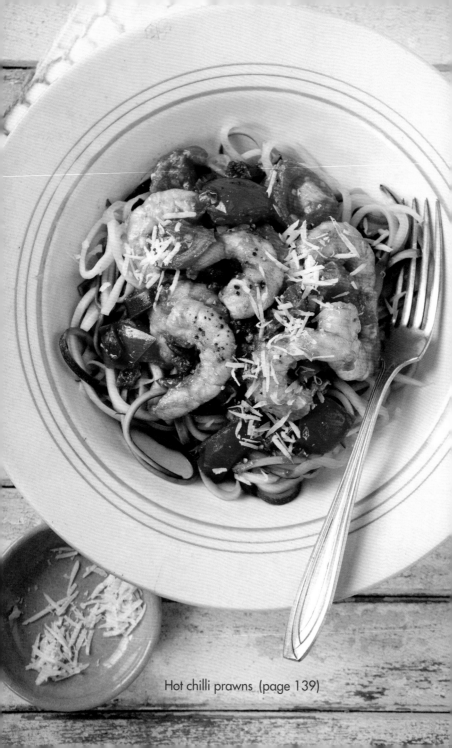

Hot chilli prawns (page 139)

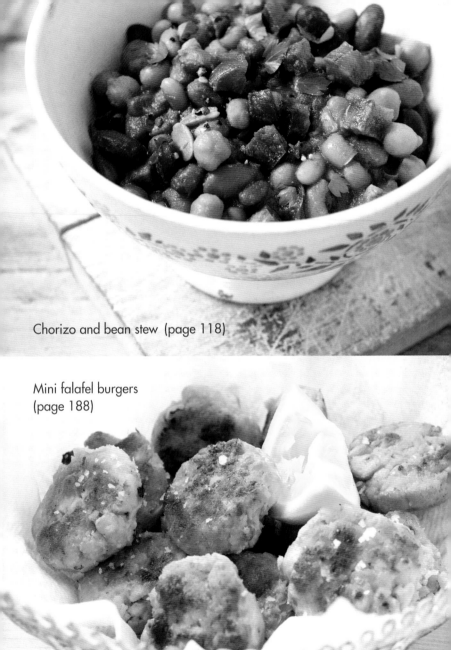

Chorizo and bean stew (page 118)

Mini falafel burgers
(page 188)

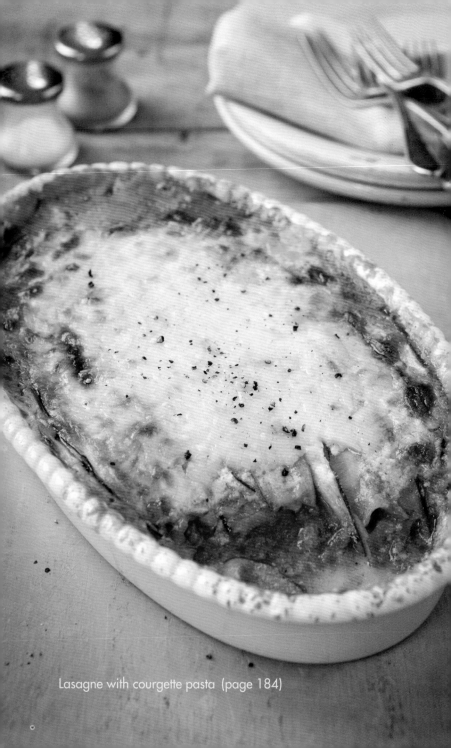

Lasagne with courgette pasta (page 184)

Orange and lemon chicken (page 158)

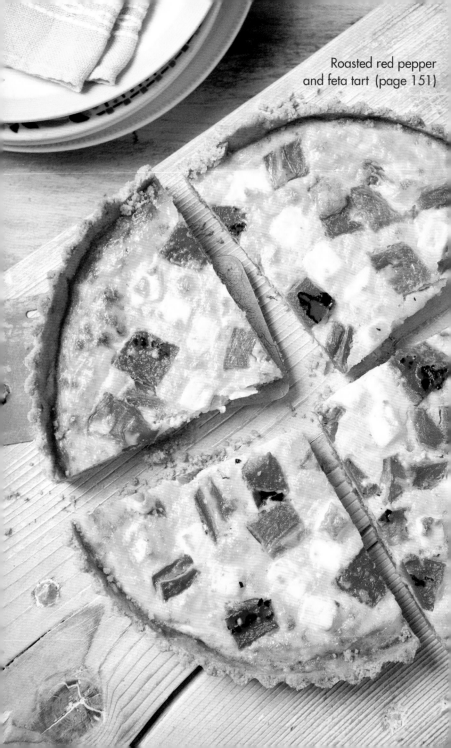

Roasted red pepper and feta tart (page 151)

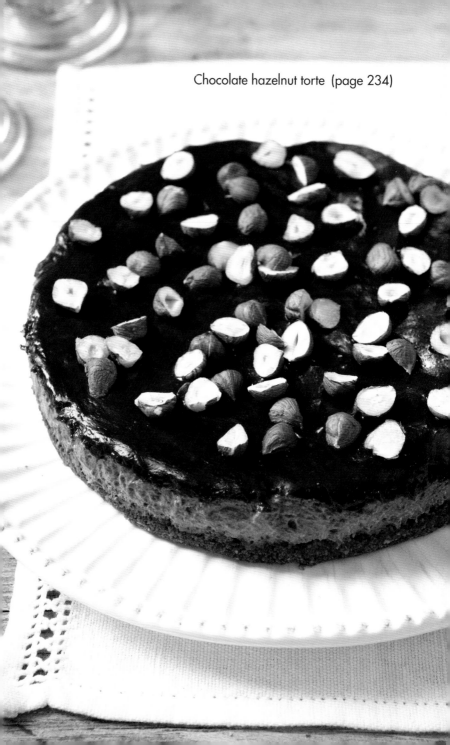

Chocolate hazelnut torte (page 234)

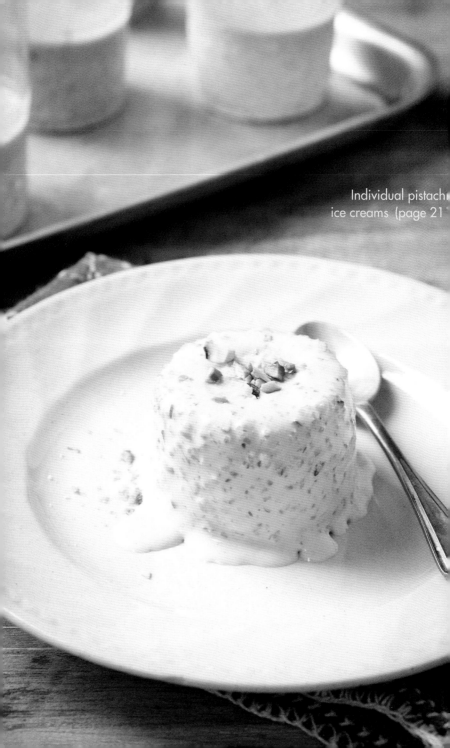

Individual pistach
ice creams (page 21

the pan. Cook for 4 minutes.

Add the cooked rice, pancetta and mushrooms to the pan. Stir together, making sure any lumps of rice are separated and heat gently until warmed through.

Quick fish fritters

A really simple way to make great tasting fishcakes.
Any white fish would work well here.

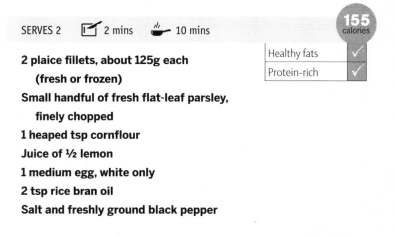

SERVES 2   2 mins   10 mins   **155** calories

Healthy fats	✓
Protein-rich	✓

2 plaice fillets, about 125g each
  (fresh or frozen)
Small handful of fresh flat-leaf parsley,
  finely chopped
1 heaped tsp cornflour
Juice of ½ lemon
1 medium egg, white only
2 tsp rice bran oil
Salt and freshly ground black pepper

Put your fish fillets in a wide pan and cover with boiling water. Cook over a high heat for 7 minutes if using fresh fish or 10 minutes if using frozen. Remove from the pan with a slotted spoon and leave to drain and cool on kitchen paper.

When the fish is cool enough to handle, use your fingers to flake the fish into a bowl, discarding any skin or bones. Add the parsley, a generous sprinkling of salt and pepper and the cornflour and toss through. Add the lemon juice and egg white and mix again. Divide the mixture into four and shape into loose patties.

Heat the oil in a heavy-based frying pan over a medium/high heat. When sizzlingly hot, gently transfer the patties to the frying pan. Fry for 2 minutes; try not to disturb them at this stage as they could break up. After 2 minutes, turn the patties over with a fish slice. Cook for a further 2 minutes. Remove from the pan, drain on kitchen paper and serve immediately.

Greek salad plate

When I want to feel a little bit special at lunchtime, I pull together some of my favourite ingredients to make this elegant yet quick dish.

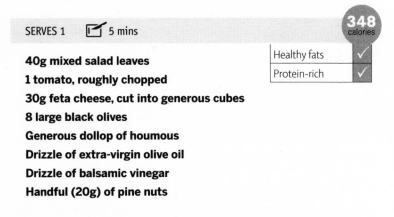

SERVES 1   5 mins

348 calories

Healthy fats	✓
Protein-rich	✓

40g mixed salad leaves
1 tomato, roughly chopped
30g feta cheese, cut into generous cubes
8 large black olives
Generous dollop of houmous
Drizzle of extra-virgin olive oil
Drizzle of balsamic vinegar
Handful (20g) of pine nuts

Take a large plate and arrange your salad leaves over one half. Arrange the tomato and feta over the leaves.

Take two very small bowls or cups (try egg cups or espresso cups) and place your olives in one and your houmous in another and place on the plate. Drizzle the olive oil and balsamic vinegar over the salad and finally scatter over the pine nuts.

Toasted cumin halloumi with butternut squash

This unusual dish has a North African feel to it, with the touch of heat tempered by the sweetness of the butternut squash and the saltiness of the halloumi.

SERVES 2   10 mins   5 mins   **285** calories

| Healthy fats | ✓ |
| Good carbs | ✓ |

300g (½ small) butternut squash, peeled and cut into large chunks

1 tsp cumin seeds

1 tsp chilli flakes

1 tbsp rapeseed oil

2 tsp tomato purée

1 tsp garlic purée (or 1 clove, crushed)

120g halloumi, cut into chunks

1 spring onion, trimmed and chopped

50g piquante peppers from a jar, drained and chopped

Juice of 1 lime

Freshly ground black pepper

Handful of fresh coriander, chopped (optional)

Place the cubed butternut squash into a microwaveable dish, cover and microwave for 5 minutes on high.

Place a frying pan over a medium/high heat and toss in the cumin seeds and chilli flakes. Dry fry for one minute, then reduce the heat to medium and add the oil, tomato purée and garlic. Stir for a few seconds before adding the halloumi and spring onions. Stir-fry for 3 minutes.

Add the peppers and butternut squash and continue to cook, stirring regularly, until browned on all sides. Remove from the heat and stir in the lime juice, black pepper and coriander. Serve immediately.

Paneer curry pot

I make this warming and filling curry pot an awful lot – it's a whole meal in a bowl. It reheats beautifully from chilled or frozen and is definitely one of those dishes you'll want to keep stacked in your freezer for a rainy day.

SERVES 4   10 mins   50 mins

377 calories

Healthy fats	✓
Good carbs	✓
Protein-rich	✓

1 tbsp rapeseed oil
1 onion, finely chopped
4 cloves garlic, finely sliced
1 large thumb-sized piece of ginger, peeled
   and cut into matchsticks
1 large chilli, seeded and cut into rings
1 red pepper, seeded and chopped
½ tsp turmeric
½ tsp cayenne pepper
1 tsp paprika
1 tsp mild chilli powder
1 tsp salt
250g puy lentils
1½ litres water, just boiled
200g peas, fresh or frozen
200g paneer, cut into cubes

2 tomatoes, roughly chopped
Juice of 1 lime

Heat the oil in a large heavy-based pan over a low heat. Add the onion, garlic, ginger, chilli and red pepper. Cook slowly for about 10 minutes until soft. Stir through the spices and salt.

Next add the puy lentils and give the mixture a really good stir. Add enough water to generously cover the lentils and bring up to a vigorous simmer. Cook on a high simmer for 10 minutes, adding more water when necessary.

Reduce the heat to very low and continue to cook for a further 20 minutes. Add more water when needed. Stir frequently to prevent it sticking to the bottom of the pan.

Add the peas, paneer and tomatoes. Cook for a further 10 minutes or until the peas are tender. Remove from the heat and stir in the lime juice. Adjust the seasoning if necessary.

Superfood salad

This delicious salad combines salmon with vegetables, nuts and seeds to get as much healthy goodness as you can in a bowl.

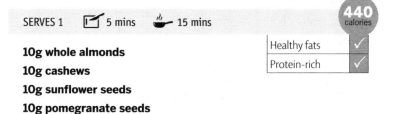

SERVES 1   5 mins   15 mins   **440** calories

| Healthy fats | ✓ |
| Protein-rich | ✓ |

10g whole almonds
10g cashews
10g sunflower seeds
10g pomegranate seeds

1 small salmon fillet (100g), skinless and boneless
2 tsp tamari (Japanese wheat-free soy sauce)
½ tsp honey
¼ tsp ground ginger
5 florets (40g) of broccoli
Handful (40g) of sugar snap peas
50g mixed salad leaves
1 fresh mint leaf, finely chopped (optional)
Small bunch (10g) of flat-leaf parsley, finely chopped (optional)
1 tomato, roughly chopped
1 spring onion, chopped

Place a small dry frying pan over a medium heat until toasty hot. Toss in the almonds, cashews and seeds. Dry fry for a few minutes, stirring frequently, until they release their aromas and start to brown. Remove from the pan and set aside.

Cut the salmon in half lengthways and add to the still hot pan. Fry the salmon in its own oil for about 4 minutes each side, until just cooked through. Remove from the pan and set aside.

Meanwhile, prepare the honey dressing for the salmon. In a shallow bowl, mix together the tamari, honey and ginger. As soon as the salmon is cool enough to handle roughly flake with your fingers into the dressing. Spoon the dressing over so that the salmon is fully covered. Leave to rest while you prepare the rest of the salad.

Simmer the broccoli and sugar snap peas together for approximately 6 minutes until tender.

Arrange the mixed leaves, herbs (if using), tomato and spring onions on a serving plate or bowl. Add the broccoli and sugar snaps. Arrange the salmon over the top and sprinkle on the nuts and seeds. Finally drizzle over any remaining dressing.

Mexican beans and cheese

These beans add a bit of pizzazz to lunchtime. As the flavour improves with time, you can leave some spare for another day; it will keep well in the fridge for 2–3 days.

SERVES 2 5 mins

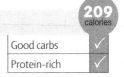
209 calories

| Good carbs | ✓ |
| Protein-rich | ✓ |

**1 x 400g tin kidney beans, rinsed
and drained**
1 tsp mild chilli powder
½ tsp ground cumin
1 tsp dried oregano
2 handfuls of crisp lettuce, such as iceberg or little gem
2 medium tomatoes, roughly chopped
40g Cheddar cheese, grated
Salt and freshly ground black pepper

Tip the drained beans into a shallow bowl and roughly mash with the back of a fork. Sprinkle over the chilli powder, cumin, oregano and a generous sprinkling of salt and pepper. Mix together until thoroughly combined.

Arrange the lettuce leaves on a plate and top with a generous serving of the beans. Add the tomatoes and finally the grated cheese.

Spanish baked prawns

I love this easy prawn dish. You can use fresh or frozen prawns so it really is a no-brainer!

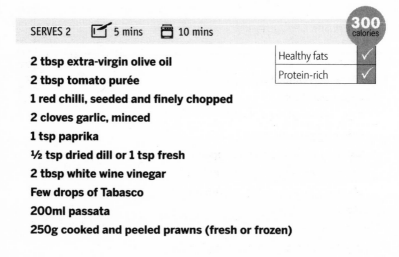

SERVES 2   5 mins   10 mins   **300** calories

2 tbsp extra-virgin olive oil
2 tbsp tomato purée
1 red chilli, seeded and finely chopped
2 cloves garlic, minced
1 tsp paprika
½ tsp dried dill or 1 tsp fresh
2 tbsp white wine vinegar
Few drops of Tabasco
200ml passata
250g cooked and peeled prawns (fresh or frozen)

| Healthy fats | ✓ |
| Protein-rich | ✓ |

Preheat the oven to 230°C/210°C fan/450°F/gas mark 8.

In a small bowl or jug mix together the olive oil, tomato purée, chilli, garlic, paprika, dill, white wine vinegar, Tabasco and passata.

Arrange the prawns in a small baking dish and pour the dressing over. Bake in the oven for 7 minutes for fresh prawns or 10 minutes for frozen.

Puy lentil and feta salad

This is an easy salad that you can put together using mainly ingredients from the store cupboard.

SERVES 2   10 mins

337 calories

Healthy fats	✓
Good carbs	✓
Protein-rich	✓

For the dressing

1 tbsp balsamic vinegar

1 tsp walnut oil

2 tsp extra-virgin olive oil

½ tsp English mustard

Salt and freshly ground pepper

1 x 400g tin ready-to-eat puy lentils, drained

30g roasted red peppers from a tin or jar, drained and chopped

30g rocket leaves

6 cherry tomatoes, halved

60g feta cheese, cut into rough cubes

30g walnuts, halved

Prepare the dressing by mixing together the balsamic vinegar, walnut oil, olive oil, English mustard and salt and pepper.

In a large bowl combine the lentils with the roasted red peppers, rocket leaves and cherry tomatoes. Stir about three-quarters of the dressing through. Arrange the feta and walnuts over the top and finally drizzle over the rest of the dressing.

Smoked salmon and cream cheese on oatcakes

This is a really simple way to get some good-quality protein and carbohydrates in a dish that takes less than 2 minutes to prepare.

SERVES 1   2 mins   **150** calories

Good carbs	✓
Protein-rich	✓

2 rough oatcakes
2 heaped tsp soft cheese
1 large slice (or 2 small) smoked salmon
½ lemon
Freshly ground black pepper

Put a spoon of soft cheese on each oatcake and roughly spread around. Arrange the salmon over the two oatcakes and squeeze a little lemon juice over each one. Finally top with a grind of black pepper.

Baked leek and blue cheese frittata

I love the way this frittata bakes so beautifully in the oven. Once you've mastered the basic technique of baking the eggs in the oven there are endless varieties you can try.

SERVES 2   5 mins   15 mins   **350** calories

Protein-rich ✓

1 tsp olive oil, for greasing
2 medium leeks, washed and sliced
75g dolcelatte (or similar blue cheese), cut into cubes
4 large eggs, lightly beaten
Salt and freshly ground black pepper

Preheat the oven to 200°C/180°C fan/400°F/gas mark 6 and place a baking sheet inside while it is preheating. Generously oil a 20cm round cake tin and line the base with a circular piece of baking parchment. Lightly oil the paper as well.

Place the leeks and 1 tablespoon of water in a small microwave-proof bowl and cover with cling film. Pierce the cling film a few times to allow the steam to escape. Cook on high in the microwave for 3 minutes.

Arrange the leeks and dolcelatte over the base of the tin and pour over the eggs. Sprinkle generously with salt and pepper.

Place the cake tin on the preheated baking sheet and bake in the oven for 15 minutes until golden brown.

Chicken Caesar salad

This is an easy salad to rustle up if you have some leftover cooked chicken.

SERVES 1   5 mins   2 mins

428 calories

Protein-rich ✓

Handful (10g) of pine nuts
2 tbsp French-style mayonnaise
1 tsp white wine vinegar
½ tsp Worcestershire sauce
1 heaped tsp capers, crushed
Freshly ground black pepper
100g cooked chicken breast, skin removed, sliced
1 Cos lettuce (60g), washed and outer leaves removed
4 large black olives
10g Parmesan cheese, finely grated

Heat a small dry frying pan over a medium/high heat. Toss in the pine nuts and cook for about 2 minutes, gently shaking the pan at intervals to make sure they're toasted all over. Transfer to a plate and leave to cool.

Combine the mayonnaise, vinegar, Worcestershire sauce, crushed capers and freshly ground black pepper in a bowl. Add the sliced chicken and mix lightly.

Arrange the lettuce on a plate and add the dressed chicken. Top with the black olives, Parmesan and toasted pine nuts.

Speedy Suppers

Courgette spaghetti

Courgette spaghetti has been a revelation to me. It's fantastically satisfying and quick to make. I don't feel tempted by pasta now because I always use this instead. You just shred a courgette with a peeler, quickly fry and serve with a sauce of your choice. I've included several of my favourite 'pasta' sauces in this chapter, all of which go beautifully with courgette spaghetti.

SERVES 1 2 mins  3 mins

63 calories

1 large courgette

Healthy fats ✓

1 tsp olive oil

Salt and freshly ground black pepper

If you want to make authentic looking spaghetti, you really need a gadget. Spiralizers are a great new kitchen accessory and are not too expensive. There is an even simpler alternative: a julienne peeler. This wasn't something I owned before but a quick look online showed me that a simple handheld peeler could be bought for under £5.

It is well worth the small outlay if you develop a taste for it. If you don't own a julienne peeler, never fear, you can use a standard vegetable peeler to create thin flat pieces of courgette. You could call this courgette tagliatelle. It tastes just as good and the preparation method is exactly the same.

Whichever type of peeler you use, start with one large washed courgette. Run the peeler down the full length of the courgette. Repeat on the same side making long pieces of courgette until you reach the seeds in the centre. Make a quarter turn in the courgette and begin again. Go all round the courgette until you have an oblong strip of seeds that can be discarded. Be careful as you near the end of the courgette as the julienne peeler is sharp and you could easily cut your finger.

Place all the peelings on a piece of kitchen paper and blot with more kitchen paper to remove the excess water.

Heat the olive oil in a wide frying pan over a high heat. Try using a flavoured oil such as garlic or chilli oil. When the oil is hot, toss in the courgette and stir. Fry for 2-3 minutes, stirring regularly. When cooked the courgette should be soft with a few browned edges. Season well with salt and pepper before serving.

Monkfish and chorizo

This dish is so quick to knock up for a one-person lunch or dinner. The flavours really pack a punch too! It works well with Courgette Spaghetti or with new potatoes and a salad.

SERVES 1   2 mins   6 mins

100g monkfish, cut into chunks
½ tsp smoked paprika
20g chorizo, finely sliced
1 tbsp dry white vermouth, such as Noilly Prat
Salt and freshly ground black pepper

Protein-rich ✓

155 calories

Place the monkfish on a small plate and sprinkle over the paprika and a little salt and pepper, then toss through.

Heat a small frying pan over a medium/high heat and add the chorizo. Fry for 2 minutes, until the oils are released and the chorizo is just starting to turn brown. Add the monkfish and fry for a further minute or two, stirring frequently until just cooked through.

Reduce the heat to low, add the vermouth and cook for 2 minutes. Serve immediately.

Creamy spicy sausage

This is a quick and flavoursome sauce using store cupboard and frozen ingredients. I love using Polish smoked kabanos in this dish but any smoked sausage would work well.
Serve with Courgette Spaghetti.

SERVES 2 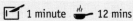 1 minute 12 mins

334 calories

100g smoked pork sausage, thinly sliced
Protein-rich ✓
150g frozen Mediterranean vegetables
  (aubergine, peppers, courgette)
1 tbsp wholegrain mustard
50ml double cream
Salt and freshly ground black pepper

Place a large non-stick frying pan over a medium heat. Fry the sausage for 3–4 minutes until just turning brown. Remove with a slotted spoon and set aside.

Add the vegetables to the frying pan, season with salt and pepper and fry over a high heat until tender, about 5 minutes. Reduce the heat to low and add two tablespoons of water. Stir in the mustard and sausage. Finally add the cream and heat through for 2 minutes until warm. Serve immediately.

Hot chilli prawns

This quick and easy sauce is a perfect accompaniment to Courgette Spaghetti.

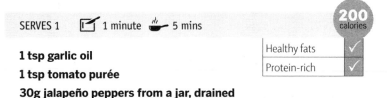

SERVES 1   1 minute   5 mins   **200** calories

| Healthy fats | ✓ |
| Protein-rich | ✓ |

1 tsp garlic oil

1 tsp tomato purée

30g jalapeño peppers from a jar, drained and chopped

2 tomatoes, chopped

100g cooked and peeled king prawns

Freshly ground black pepper

10g Parmesan, finely grated

Heat the garlic oil in a frying pan over a medium heat and fry the tomato purée for a minute before adding the jalapeños and chopped tomatoes. Fry for 2–3 minutes, until the tomatoes start to soften.

Add the prawns and warm through for a couple of minutes. Season generously with black pepper and serve immediately, sprinkled with the grated Parmesan.

Sun-dried tomato and cashew nut

If you've not got much time, this is the ultimate store cupboard saviour.

SERVES 1   1 minute   **295** calories

Protein-rich ✓

30g sun-dried tomatoes in oil, drained
30g feta cheese, cubed
20g cashew nuts

Simply mix all the ingredients in with your just cooked Courgette Spaghetti and warm through.

Warm prawn and avocado salad

Puy lentils add a complex earthiness to this dish. They contain the best kind of carbohydrates plus protein and fibre. Best of all, they can be bought pre-cooked and are ready to eat in a jiffy.

SERVES 2   10 minute   3 mins   **368** calories

Good carbs ✓
Protein-rich ✓

200g cooked king prawns
1 red chilli, seeded and finely chopped
Zest and juice of 1 lime
1 tbsp light soy sauce
1 tsp clear honey
½ x 400g tin puy lentils, drained

1 avocado, peeled, stoned and sliced

4 radishes, washed, trimmed and finely sliced

Handful of fresh coriander, finely chopped (optional)

1 tsp sesame oil

2 pak choi, separated into leaves and ends removed

Place the prawns in a bowl with the chilli, lime zest and half the lime juice. Mix together and set aside while you prepare the rest of the dish.

In a small bowl, mix together the soy sauce, honey and the rest of the lime juice. Put the lentils, avocado, radishes and coriander, if using, in a large bowl and stir through the soy dressing.

Heat the sesame oil in a frying pan and toss in the pak choi. Fry over a high heat until just wilted. Add the prawns and their marinade and warm through for 1–2 minutes.

Divide the lentil salad between two plates and put the prawns and pak choi on top. Serve immediately.

Parmesan chicken

This is a deliciously easy way to cook chicken, and it's great for both kids and adults. I like to serve it with new potatoes and peas.

SERVES 2   4 mins   10 mins   **425** calories

Protein-rich ✓

2 tbsp gram (chickpea) flour
1 egg, lightly beaten
30g Parmesan, finely grated
2 chicken breasts, each cut into 4–5 strips
1–2 tbsp olive oil
Salt and freshly ground black pepper

Place the gram flour, egg and Parmesan in three separate shallow bowls, adding salt and pepper to the Parmesan bowl.

Prepare the chicken by dipping each piece first in the flour, then the egg and finally the Parmesan.

Heat the oil in a large frying pan over a medium heat. Place the chicken strips in the pan, leaving as much space as possible between the pieces. Cook for 3–5 minutes each side until brown, crunchy and cooked through. Serve immediately.

Mushroom stroganoff

This fab midweek supper is easy and filling.

SERVES 1   10 mins (including soaking time)   10 mins   **160** calories

3 dried porcini mushrooms (about 1g)
1 tsp olive oil
1 spring onion, chopped
1 clove garlic, finely chopped
250g mushrooms, sliced
1 tbsp cooking sherry or similar
1 tsp paprika
1 tsp Dijon mustard
1 tsp cornflour
100ml water
1 heaped tbsp Greek yoghurt
Salt and freshly ground black pepper

Healthy fats	✓
Probiotics	✓

Place the porcini mushrooms in a small bowl and pour over about 100ml of boiling water. Leave to soak for 10 minutes.

Meanwhile, heat the oil in a wide frying pan over a medium heat and toss in the spring onion, garlic and mushrooms. Turn the heat to high and fry for 2–4 minutes, until tender and glossy.

Reduce the heat and splash in the sherry. Stir in the paprika, Dijon mustard and cornflour. Slowly add the water, stirring continuously, until the sauce starts to thicken. Chop the soaked porcini mushrooms and add to the pan along with their soaking liquor (strain it first to remove the bits at the bottom of the bowl.

Bring to a simmer and cook for 7 minutes. Season to taste with salt and pepper and then remove from the heat and stir in the Greek yoghurt just before serving.

Hot steak fajitas

Home-made fajitas are so easy. I never understand why you would need a kit for this! Serve with a green salad, grated cheese, natural yoghurt and home-made salsa. You can buy wheat-free corn tortillas from the specialist aisle of the supermarket or make your own (page 109).

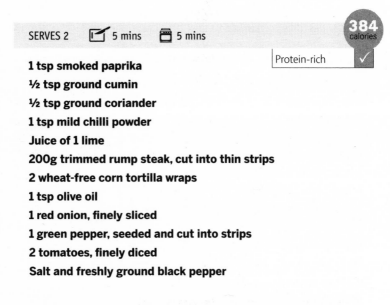

SERVES 2   5 mins   5 mins

384 calories

Protein-rich ✓

1 tsp smoked paprika
½ tsp ground cumin
½ tsp ground coriander
1 tsp mild chilli powder
Juice of 1 lime
200g trimmed rump steak, cut into thin strips
2 wheat-free corn tortilla wraps
1 tsp olive oil
1 red onion, finely sliced
1 green pepper, seeded and cut into strips
2 tomatoes, finely diced
Salt and freshly ground black pepper

Preheat the oven to 200°C/180°C fan/400°F/gas mark 6.

Mix the spices, lime juice and salt and pepper in a large bowl. Add the steak strips and mix together thoroughly with your hands. Leave to stand for a few minutes while you prepare the rest of the meal.

Wrap the tortillas in foil and warm through in the oven for about 5 minutes.

Heat the olive oil in a large non-stick frying pan over a high heat. When hot, toss in the onion and green pepper and fry for 2 minutes. Add the steak strips and any reserved marinade and cook for 2-3 minutes, stirring once. Stir in the chopped tomato and cook for a further minute.

Serve with the warmed tortillas directly from the foil.

Egg florentine

A poached egg with hollandaise sauce is a perfect easy meal for one. I use a quick 'cheats' hollandaise here.

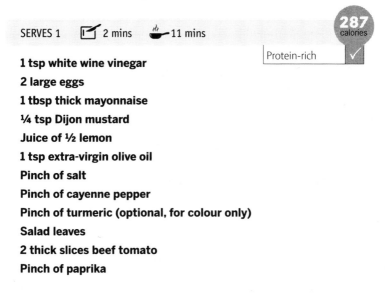

SERVES 1   2 mins   11 mins   287 calories

Protein-rich ✓

1 tsp white wine vinegar
2 large eggs
1 tbsp thick mayonnaise
¼ tsp Dijon mustard
Juice of ½ lemon
1 tsp extra-virgin olive oil
Pinch of salt
Pinch of cayenne pepper
Pinch of turmeric (optional, for colour only)
Salad leaves
2 thick slices beef tomato
Pinch of paprika

Fill a wide pan with 4-5cm water. Bring up to simmering point and then add the vinegar. The water should be just simmering with a few occasional bubbles.

Crack the first egg on the side of the pan and then gently lower it into the water. Repeat with the second egg. Simmer for exactly 1 minute before turning the heat off and leaving the eggs to cook in the slowly cooling water for a further 10 minutes. This should ensure a cooked egg with a runny middle.

Meanwhile prepare the mock hollandaise. Put the mayonnaise, mustard, lemon juice, olive oil, salt, cayenne pepper and turmeric in a small bowl or jug and whisk together until smooth.

Arrange the salad leaves on a plate and add the tomato slices. Then, using a slotted spoon, carefully transfer the eggs to the top of each tomato slice. Pour over the hollandaise sauce and top with a pinch of paprika.

Delicious Dinners

Mediterranean lamb stew

This simple dish is very flavoursome and makes a great summer stew. I like to incorporate the potatoes in the dish to make a complete meal but they can be left out if you prefer.

SERVES 4   10 mins   1½ hours   **575** calories

| Good carbs | ✓ |
| Protein-rich | ✓ |

1 large onion, chopped

600g diced lamb

600g fresh tomatoes, roughly chopped

400g new potatoes, halved

Zest and juice of ½ orange

2 tsp cumin seeds

200ml chicken stock, warmed

1 tbsp tomato purée

Pinch of sugar

2 bay leaves

Salt and freshly ground black pepper

Preheat the oven to 210°C/190°C fan/400°F/gas mark 6.

Arrange the onion over the base of a deep baking dish. Add the lamb, tomatoes and new potatoes. Sprinkle over the orange zest and juice.

Crush the cumin seeds lightly in a pestle and mortar and sprinkle over the lamb. Dissolve the tomato purée and sugar in the chicken stock and pour over the lamb. Tuck in the bay leaves and season generously with salt and pepper. Cover with foil and bake in the oven for 1½ hours, or until the meat is very tender.

Sesame chicken noodles

In this recipe we use a julienne peeler or spiralizer (page 136) to create cucumber 'noodles'. Or if you don't have either of those, use a normal vegetable peeler to make thick ribbons of cucumber.

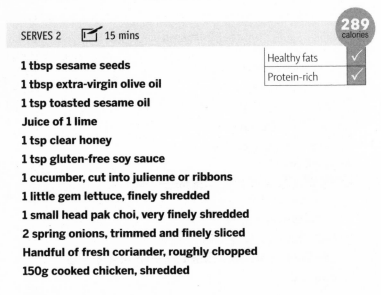

SERVES 2   15 mins   **289** calories

Healthy fats	✓
Protein-rich	✓

1 tbsp sesame seeds
1 tbsp extra-virgin olive oil
1 tsp toasted sesame oil
Juice of 1 lime
1 tsp clear honey
1 tsp gluten-free soy sauce
1 cucumber, cut into julienne or ribbons
1 little gem lettuce, finely shredded
1 small head pak choi, very finely shredded
2 spring onions, trimmed and finely sliced
Handful of fresh coriander, roughly chopped
150g cooked chicken, shredded

Toast the sesame seeds in a small dry frying pan for 2 minutes, until lightly browned and fragrant. Transfer to a plate to cool.

In a small bowl, mix together the olive oil, sesame oil, lime juice, honey and soy sauce.

Place the cucumber, lettuce, pak choi, spring onions and coriander in a large bowl and gently mix together. Pour over the dressing and mix again.

Distribute the salad between two plates and top with the shredded chicken. Sprinkle over the sesame seeds just before serving.

Roasted red pepper and feta tart

The crust on this tart tastes amazing; it has just the right amount of crunch and crumble so that you'd struggle to tell the difference between this and shortcrust pastry. Even better, there's no rolling involved.

SERVES 4   15 mins   20 mins   28 mins   **434** calories

Protein-rich ✓

100g ground almonds
50g gram (chickpea) flour
½ tsp bicarbonate of soda
pinch of salt
60g butter, melted, plus extra for greasing
2 large eggs
30g Cheddar, grated
2 tbsp natural yoghurt
**50g roasted red peppers from a jar, drained and roughly
  chopped**

Few sprigs of fresh oregano, chopped or ½ tsp dried
50g feta, cubed
Freshly ground black pepper

Lightly grease a 20cm loose-bottomed cake tin and set aside.

Place the ground almonds, gram flour, bicarbonate of soda and salt in a large bowl and mix gently. Pour in the melted butter and stir to combine until you have a firm dough.

Scoop three-quarters of the dough into the tin and press down firmly into the base. Distribute the rest of the dough mix around the edges of the tin and press into the sides, making a lip about 2cm high. Make sure you don't have any gaps in the pastry and it is evenly distributed. Place the tin in the fridge for about 20 minutes to chill.

Preheat the oven to 210°C/190°C fan/425°F/gas mark 7. Use a fork to prick several shallow holes in the base of the pastry and then bake in the oven for 10 minutes, until golden brown. Remove from the and set aside. Reduce the oven temperature to 190°C/170°C fan/375°F/gas mark 5.

Crack the eggs into a bowl and beat well. Add the grated cheese, yoghurt, red peppers and oregano. Mix well and pour into the pastry. Dot the cubed feta evenly around the tart and sprinkle over a little black pepper.

Bake for 18–20 minutes, or until the filling is just set and turning golden brown. Remove from the oven and leave to cool in the tin for 10 minutes. This tart can be served hot or cold.

Pad thai

This amazing recipe uses shirataki noodles. Made from Japanese yam, they are naturally low in carbohydrate and can be used in any recipe requiring thin rice noodles. Although these are increasingly found in large supermarkets and health food shops, the best place to buy them is a Chinese supermarket.

SERVES 2 10 mins 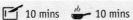 10 mins **363** calories

Protein-rich ✓

1 tsp brown sugar

Juice of 1 lime

200g chicken breast, thinly sliced

1 tbsp rice wine vinegar

1 tbsp water

1 tbsp gluten-free soy sauce

1 tbsp fish sauce

2 large eggs

Pinch of salt

2 tbsp rice bran oil

1 chilli, seeded and diced

1 clove garlic, finely chopped

1 small thumb-sized piece of ginger, peeled and cut into thin matchsticks

3 spring onions, trimmed and sliced

170g shirataki noodles, soaked in warm water and drained

½ carrot, peeled and grated

100g beansprouts

Handful of fresh coriander, chopped

Extra lime wedges, to serve

Place the brown sugar and lime juice in a bowl and toss in the sliced chicken. Mix it all together and set aside to rest.

In a small dish mix together the rice wine vinegar, water, soy and fish sauces. In a separate bowl, whisk the eggs lightly with the salt.

Heat the rice bran oil in a wok or large frying pan over a high heat. Add the chilli, garlic, ginger and half the spring onions and fry for 1 minute before tossing in the chicken, together with its marinade. Stir-fry until the chicken is nearly cooked. Pour in the beaten eggs and let it cook until the egg mixture sets around the chicken and the chicken is cooked through. Then break up the egg by stirring thoroughly; transfer the eggs and chicken to a plate.

Return the wok to the heat and toss in the drained noodles. Stir-fry for several minutes until they are bone dry. Move the noodles around to form a well in the centre and add the grated carrot, beansprouts and remaining spring onions. Stir-fry for another couple of minutes, stirring and pressing the mixture down against the bottom of the wok. Add the soy sauce mixture and stir through for a minute or two before adding the chicken and egg mixture. Stir for another minute before adding the coriander. Serve immediately with a wedge of lime on the side.

Lentil and mushroom bolognaise

This bolognaise is so filling and versatile that you simply don't need the meat. There is enough here to serve 6 but it freezes well so you can freeze individual portions. Simply re-heat in the microwave for a delicious sauce in seconds. Serve over Courgette Spaghetti (page 135) or half a baked potato.

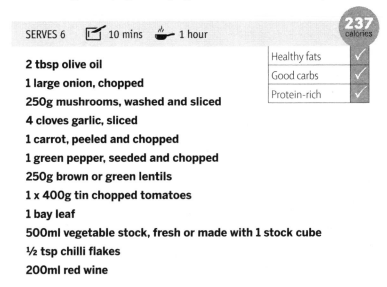

SERVES 6 | 10 mins | 1 hour

237 calories

Healthy fats	✓
Good carbs	✓
Protein-rich	✓

2 tbsp olive oil

1 large onion, chopped

250g mushrooms, washed and sliced

4 cloves garlic, sliced

1 carrot, peeled and chopped

1 green pepper, seeded and chopped

250g brown or green lentils

1 x 400g tin chopped tomatoes

1 bay leaf

500ml vegetable stock, fresh or made with 1 stock cube

½ tsp chilli flakes

200ml red wine

In a large pan, heat the oil over a medium heat. Fry the onion for 5 minutes. Add the mushrooms, garlic, carrot and green pepper. Cook for 15-20 minutes until soft, stirring frequently.

Stir in the lentils, then add the chopped tomatoes, bay leaf, vegetable stock and chilli flakes. Bring to the boil and cook on a vigorous heat for 10 minutes. Reduce the heat to medium/low, add the wine and cook for a further 20-30 minutes until the sauce is rich and thick.

Beef curry

There are a lot of ingredients in this recipe but this amazing curry is definitely worth the effort.

SERVES 2　　　📠 20 mins　　🍲 2 hours 40 mins　　**482** calories

Protein-rich　✓

250g cooked beetroot, drained or
　vacuum-packed
2.5-cm piece of ginger, peeled and roughly chopped
1 clove garlic
1 red chilli, seeded
2 cardamom pods
1 tbsp tomato purée
1 heaped tsp black treacle
1 tsp ground cumin
1 tsp ground coriander
1 tsp fennel seeds
1 tsp mild chilli powder
Pinch of ground cloves
½ tsp black pepper
1 tbsp rapeseed oil
300g stewing steak, diced
1 onion, chopped
1 green pepper, seeded and chopped
Pinch of salt
500ml water
½ tsp garam masala
Handful of fresh coriander, chopped

Put one of the beetroots in a blender or food processor. Add the ginger, garlic, chilli, cardamom pods, tomato purée, treacle, all the spices and the black pepper. Whizz to smooth paste, adding a little water to loosen if necessary.

Heat the oil over a high heat in a flameproof casserole dish. Fry the beef until browned all over. Transfer to a dish with a slotted spoon and set aside.

Reduce the heat and toss in the onion, green pepper and salt. Fry gently for 5 minutes before adding the beetroot and spice paste. Stir through and fry for 2–3 minutes.

Roughly chop the remaining beetroot and add to the pan. Add the beef and water to the pan, stir thoroughly and bring to the boil. Simmer on the hob for about 30 minutes. Meanwhile preheat the oven to 160°C/140°C fan/325°F/gas mark 3.

Place the lid on the pan and transfer to the oven. Cook for 2 hours. Alternatively, you could transfer to a slow cooker and cook for 6–8 hours.

Stir through the garam masala and then taste and adjust the seasoning. Scatter with chopped fresh coriander before serving.

Orange and lemon chicken

This is a simple but zesty chicken dish. Serve with new potatoes and a green vegetable such as broccoli or sugar snap peas.

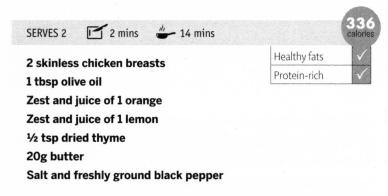

SERVES 2   2 mins   14 mins   **336** calories

2 skinless chicken breasts
1 tbsp olive oil
Zest and juice of 1 orange
Zest and juice of 1 lemon
½ tsp dried thyme
20g butter
Salt and freshly ground black pepper

| Healthy fats | ✓ |
| Protein-rich | ✓ |

Cut the chicken breasts in half widthways, making two fat pieces. Make a cut about 2.5cm long into the thickest part of each chicken piece. This flattens the chicken slightly, allowing it to cook quicker and makes a simple butterfly shape.

Heat the oil in a frying pan over a medium/high heat. When hot, add the chicken pieces. Sprinkle over the orange and lemon zest and the thyme and season well with salt and pepper. Cook for 3–4 minutes on each side, until golden and just cooked through.

Add the orange and juices to the pan and allow to sizzle. Reduce the heat to low and let the sauce bubble for 2 minutes. Transfer the chicken to a warm plate.

Add the butter to the pan and cook over a high heat for 2–4 minutes, until you have a thick glossy sauce. Pour over the chicken and serve immediately.

White fish with pesto crust

Make a rustic-style pesto and use it to top a piece of white fish. This is a very pleasing and quick-to-serve dish that can be made with haddock, cod, sea bass or any similar white fish.

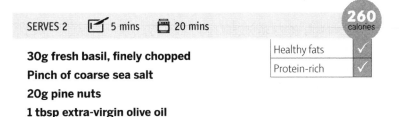

SERVES 2   5 mins   20 mins   **260** calories

30g fresh basil, finely chopped
Pinch of coarse sea salt
20g pine nuts
1 tbsp extra-virgin olive oil
10g Parmesan, finely grated
Freshly ground black pepper
2 x 150-g skinless fish fillets

| Healthy fats | ✓ |
| Protein-rich | ✓ |

Preheat the oven to 200°C/180°C fan/400°F/gas mark 6.

Place the basil in a pestle and mortar with the sea salt and grind until you get a mushy paste. Add the pine nuts and grind again. Add the olive oil, Parmesan and black pepper. Stir together.

Place the fish on a baking tray and divide the pesto between the fish pieces. Spread the pesto so that it covers the top of both fillets evenly. Bake in the oven for 15–20 minutes, depending on the size and shape of the fish.

Thai vegetable curry

*This sweet and colourful curry is a firm favourite
in our house.*

SERVES 2   20 mins   20 mins

308 calories

**300g butternut squash (½ to 1 small),
     peeled, seeded and cut into small chunks**

4 tsp olive oil

2 tbsp desiccated coconut

1 tsp cumin seeds

2 spring onions, trimmed and chopped

1 red chilli, seeded and finely chopped

1 thumb-sized piece of ginger, peeled and finely grated

1 tsp lemongrass paste

100g baby corn

100g mangetout

2 basil leaves, chopped

Juice of 1 lime

170g Greek yoghurt

Salt

Healthy fats	✓
Good carbs	✓
Probiotics	✓

Preheat the oven to 220°C/200°C fan/425°F/gas mark 7.

Arrange the squash chunks in a roasting tin and pour over
3 teaspoons of the olive oil. Toss through with your hands until
evenly coated. Roast for 15–20 minutes until just tender.

Meanwhile, place the coconut and cumin seeds in a pestle and
mortar and crush until the coconut is about half its original size.

Heat the remaining teaspoon of olive oil in a deep, lidded frying
pan and toss in the spring onions and chilli. Fry lightly for about 2

minutes before adding the ginger, lemongrass, coconut paste and about a tablespoon of water. Stir well before adding the baby corn and mangetout. Reduce the heat to its lowest setting, place the lid on the pan and cook for 6–8 minutes, or until the vegetables are just tender.

Remove the lid from the pan and add the cooked butternut squash, basil, lime juice and 3–4 tablespoons water. Stir through and cook for a couple of minutes until hot through. Check the seasoning and add a little salt if necessary.

Remove the pan from the heat (this is necessary as the cultures in the natural yoghurt would be destroyed with cooking). Add the yoghurt and stir through, adding a little more water if required. Serve immediately.

Turkish kofta kebabs

These are perfect for the barbecue but can also be cooked on a griddle pan or under the grill.

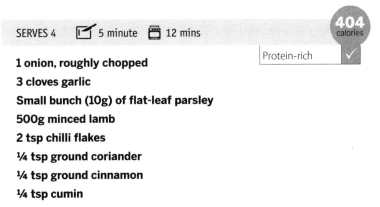

SERVES 4   5 minute   12 mins   **404** calories

Protein-rich ✓

1 onion, roughly chopped
3 cloves garlic
Small bunch (10g) of flat-leaf parsley
500g minced lamb
2 tsp chilli flakes
¼ tsp ground coriander
¼ tsp ground cinnamon
¼ tsp cumin

1 tbsp rapeseed oil
Salt and freshly ground black pepper

Cover 4 wooden skewers with cold water and leave to soak. Heat up your barbecue or grill to a high temperature.

Blitz the onion, garlic and parsley in a food processor until finely chopped (you can also do this by hand).

Place the lamb, onion and garlic paste, chilli flakes and spices in a large bowl. Season generously with salt and pepper. Use your hands to mash and knead the meat until the individual strands of mince disappear and everything is really well combined.

Divide the mixture into four and mould it into sausage shapes around the skewers.

Brush the kofta with the oil. Cook on the barbecue, grill or griddle for between 8–12 minutes, turning regularly, until browned and cooked through.

Fresh saag paneer

Using fresh spinach in this recipe gives the dish more zing. It's lighter and fresher than the version served in most curry houses.

SERVES 4   10 mins   30 mins   **176** calories

Protein-rich ✓

1 tbsp rice bran oil
250g paneer, cut into cubes
1 onion, chopped
1 thumb-sized piece of ginger, peeled and cut into matchsticks

2 cloves garlic, finely sliced

1 fresh green chilli, seeded and cut into rings

1 tsp tomato purée

200g cherry tomatoes, halved

1 tsp ground coriander

1 tsp ground cumin

¼ tsp ground turmeric

1 tsp mild chilli powder

200g fresh spinach leaves

Salt and freshly ground black pepper

Heat the oil in a wide, lidded frying pan over a high heat. Add the paneer cubes and season generously with salt and pepper. Fry for a few minutes until golden, stirring often. Remove from the pan and set aside.

Reduce the heat and add the onion. Fry for 5 minutes before adding the ginger, garlic and chilli. Fry for another 5 minutes. Add the tomato purée and cherry tomatoes. Put the lid on the pan and cook for a further 5–7 minutes.

Add all the spices and a little more salt. Return the paneer to the pan and stir until coated. Then add the spinach leaves and return the lid to the pan. Allow the spinach to wilt for 2–3 minutes and then stir into the sauce.

Piri piri chicken

A delicious spicy marinade for your chicken. I use two bird's eye chillies here, which gives it quite a kick. Feel free to adjust up or down depending on how hot you like it. For an authentic taste the chicken should be marinated overnight and cooked on a barbecue.

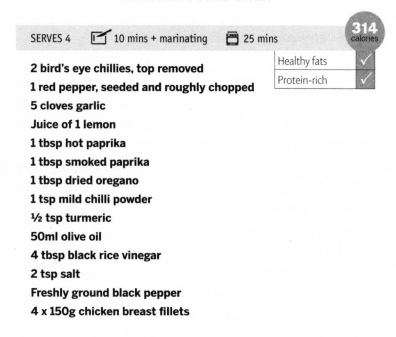

SERVES 4   10 mins + marinating   25 mins   **314** calories

Healthy fats	✓
Protein-rich	✓

2 bird's eye chillies, top removed

1 red pepper, seeded and roughly chopped

5 cloves garlic

Juice of 1 lemon

1 tbsp hot paprika

1 tbsp smoked paprika

1 tbsp dried oregano

1 tsp mild chilli powder

½ tsp turmeric

50ml olive oil

4 tbsp black rice vinegar

2 tsp salt

Freshly ground black pepper

4 x 150g chicken breast fillets

Place the chillies, red pepper and garlic in a food processor or blender and blitz until finely chopped. Add the lemon juice, spices, salt, olive oil, vinegar, salt and black pepper. Blend again until you have a smooth paste.

Cut the chicken breasts in half widthways, making two fat pieces. Make a cut about 2.5cm long into the thickest part of each chicken piece. This flattens the chicken slightly allowing it to cook quicker and makes a simple butterfly shape. Place the chicken in a bowl and pour over the marinade. Rub the marinade all over the chicken, then cover and refrigerate overnight.

Preheat the oven to 190°C/170°C fan/375°F/gas mark 5.

Heat a wide, heavy-based frying pan to a very high temperature. Shake off the excess marinade and place in the hot pan. Cook for 2 minutes each side, just to seal the chicken pieces rather than cook them right through.

Arrange the chicken pieces on a baking tray and pop in the oven for 10 minutes. Remove from the oven and smooth over a little more marinade. Reduce the oven temperature to 140°C/120°C fan/275°/gas mark 1 and cook for a further 10 minutes, or until cooked through.

Place the remaining marinade in a small pan with about 100ml water and simmer for about 5–10 minutes until thickened. Serve the chicken with the sauce on the side and a crisp salad.

Moroccan chickpea stew

This unusual and earthy Moroccan stew is a warming winter dish which works equally well as a main meal or as a 'tupperware lunch', to be heated in the office microwave.

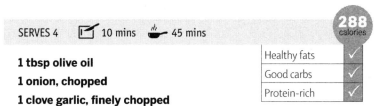

SERVES 4   10 mins   45 mins   **288** calories

1 tbsp olive oil
1 onion, chopped
1 clove garlic, finely chopped

Healthy fats	✓
Good carbs	✓
Protein-rich	✓

1 red pepper, seeded and diced
1 aubergine, cut into chunks
2 tsp ground cumin
½ tsp ground cinnamon
2 tsp ground coriander
1 tbsp tomato purée
2 tbsp harissa paste
1 x 400g tin chickpeas, rinsed and drained
150g red lentils
20g fresh flat-leaf parsley
2 tomatoes, roughly chopped
Juice of 1 lemon
Salt and freshly ground black pepper

Heat the oil in a large pan, add the onion and fry for 7–8 minutes until translucent. Add the garlic, pepper and aubergine and fry for another 5 minutes. Add in the spices, tomato purée and harissa paste and stir through for a minute or two.

Add the chickpeas and lentils and cover generously with 800–900ml of just-boiled water. Bring to the boil and simmer vigorously for 10 minutes. Then reduce the heat and simmer gently for a further 15 minutes. Keep topping up the water if it threatens to dry out.

Remove from the heat and stir in the parsley, tomatoes and lemon juice. Season with salt and pepper and serve immediately.

Oriental salmon fishcakes

These elegant, oriental-style fishcakes are a bit different from the norm.

SERVES 2   5 mins   6 mins   **462** calories

| Healthy fats | ✓ |
| Protein-rich | ✓ |

2 skinless salmon fillets (approximately 130g each), cut into chunks
2 spring onions, chopped
1 small egg, beaten
2 heaped tbsp gram (chickpea) flour
1 tbsp desiccated coconut
½ tsp nam pla fish sauce
Small handful of fresh coriander, roughly chopped
Juice of ½ lime
2 tbsp rice bran oil
Lime wedges, to serve

Place the salmon in a food processor and pulse briefly. Add the spring onions, egg, gram flour, coconut, fish sauce, coriander and lime juice to the salmon and blitz again until roughly combined.

Heat the oil in a heavy-based frying pan and when hot add tablespoons of the salmon mixture to the pan. Press down lightly on the top of the salmon to make them into patties no more than 1cm thick. Cook for 2–3 minutes each side and turn gently with a fish slice. Be careful as they can be delicate.

Serve with a wedge of lime on the side.

10

Family Favourites

Moussaka

My children love the sweet yet sophisticated taste of the lightly spiced lamb. They don't even notice the aubergine. Definitely a win-win for me. An extra advantage is that the topping is simply made from Greek yoghurt and egg, no whisking required. The moussaka can be made in advance, frozen and cooked straight from the freezer. Simply add an extra 30 minutes to the cooking time.

SERVES 4   20 mins   1½ hours   **560** calories

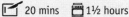 Good carbs ✓

1 tbsp olive oil

1 large onion, finely chopped

1 green pepper, seeded and chopped

400g lamb mince

1 courgette, trimmed and roughly diced

2 cloves garlic, thinly sliced

½ tsp cinnamon

¼ tsp nutmeg
¼ tsp ground cloves
1 x 400g tin chopped tomatoes
2 bay leaves
1 tsp dried thyme
½ tsp dried oregano
1 large or 2 small aubergines
200g Greek yoghurt
1 large egg
1 tbsp cream cheese
50g Parmesan, finely grated
50g mature Cheddar, grated
Salt and freshly ground black pepper

In a large pan, heat the olive oil over a low heat. Add the onions and green pepper and fry for 5 minutes. Turn the heat up to high and crumble in the lamb mince with your fingers. Stir-fry the mince until just browned, making sure you break up any large clumps of meat with the back of the spoon.

Reduce the heat to low and add the courgette, garlic and spices. Stir through before adding the chopped tomatoes, bay leaves and dried herbs. Season with salt and pepper. Bring up to simmering point before leaving to bubble gently for about 30 minutes.

Preheat the oven to 180°C/160°C fan/350°F/gas mark 4.

Meanwhile, prepare the aubergines and cheese sauce. There is no need to salt the aubergines for this dish as they will soak up the lovely flavour of the sauce. Simply wash and cut into thin slices about 3–5mm thick. To make the cheese sauce, place the Greek yoghurt in a bowl and whisk in the egg with a fork. Stir in the cream cheese. Set aside about a quarter of both the Parmesan and Cheddar cheeses and mix the rest into the yoghurt.

Cover the base of a large ovenproof dish with about half of the mince and arrange half of the aubergine slices over the top. Add a smaller portion of mince and arrange the rest of the aubergine slices over the top of that. Finish off with the remaining mince and spread the cheese sauce over the top.

Bake in the preheated oven for 40-45 minutes until bubbling and golden. Remove from the oven and leave to rest for 5-10 minutes before serving with a simple salad.

Easy tomato sauce

This delicious tomato sauce is great as a topping for Courgette Spaghetti (page 135) or with the All-you-can-eat Pizza (page 172).

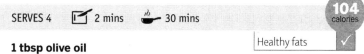

SERVES 4 2 mins 30 mins **104** calories

Healthy fats ✓

1 tbsp olive oil
1 onion, finely chopped
3 cloves garlic, finely sliced
125ml white wine
500ml passata
Handful of fresh basil, chopped
Salt and freshly ground black pepper

Heat the olive oil in a deep frying pan and add the onion and garlic. Fry gently for 5 minutes until softened. Turn the heat up and add the white wine. Let it bubble for 2-3 minutes.

Add the passata, basil and season generously with salt and

pepper. Simmer for about 30 minutes until reduced to a thick sauce.

This sauce can be kept in the fridge for up to 3 days or frozen for a later date.

All-you-can-eat pizza

Wheat-free pizza is never going to be quite the same as a wheat-based variety. But this new recipe is totally yummy and easy to make. Top with tomato sauce and your favourite toppings.

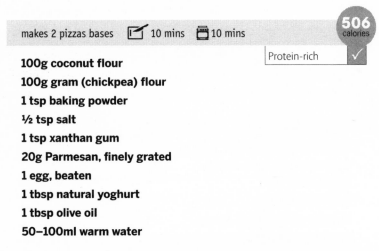

makes 2 pizzas bases   10 mins   10 mins   **506** calories

Protein-rich ✓

100g coconut flour
100g gram (chickpea) flour
1 tsp baking powder
½ tsp salt
1 tsp xanthan gum
20g Parmesan, finely grated
1 egg, beaten
1 tbsp natural yoghurt
1 tbsp olive oil
50–100ml warm water

Mix the coconut flour, gram flour, baking powder, salt, xanthan gum and Parmesan together in a bowl. Add the beaten egg, natural yoghurt and olive oil. Slowly add the water, bringing the dough together with your hands. There is enough water when the dough is soft and pliable and a little wet.

Knead lightly with your hands and divide into two equal balls. Roll the balls between your hands so they are smooth. Place one ball on a large piece of baking parchment and use a piece of cling film on the top to roll out into a roughly circular shape about 20cm in diameter and about 5mm thick. Remove the cling film before cutting round the edges of the pizza, using a cake tin or similar as a guide.

Place the dough, still on the baking parchment, in the microwave and cook on high for 2 minutes. Turn the pizza over and keep pliable by wrapping immediately in a tea towel. Repeat with the other pizza base.

Preheat the oven to 220°C/200°C fan/425°F/gas mark 7. Top the pizza bases with tomato sauce (page 171), mozzarella cheese and your favourite toppings before baking in the oven for about 10 minutes.

Sweet and sour chicken

An easy, everyday supper. Serve with brown rice.

SERVES 2   5 mins   9 mins   **319** calories

2 skinless chicken breasts, cut into strips

| Healthy fats | ✓ |
| Protein-rich | ✓ |

1 small onion, sliced

1 red pepper, seeded and sliced

½ head broccoli, cut into small florets

1 clove garlic, finely sliced

2 tsp cornflour

1 tbsp olive oil

1 tsp clear honey

1 tbsp white wine vinegar

1 tsp tomato purée

1 tsp soy sauce

½ tsp English mustard

50ml water

1 tbsp dry (not cream) sherry

Salt and freshly ground black pepper

Place the chicken, onion, pepper, broccoli and garlic in a bowl. Sprinkle over the cornflour and season with salt and pepper. Mix together thoroughly.

Heat the oil in a wide pan over a medium heat. Toss in the chicken and vegetable mixture and cook, stirring every minute, until just cooked (about 5–7 minutes, depending on size).

Meanwhile mix the honey, vinegar, tomato purée, soy sauce, English mustard, water and sherry in a small bowl. When the chicken is just cooked, stir in the sauce and allow to bubble gently for 2 minutes before serving.

Sausage hotpot

This is a very comforting, all-in-one dish.

SERVES 4　　5 mins　　1½ hours　　**462** calories

Good carbs	✓
Protein-rich	✓

600g new potatoes, skin on

6 large gluten-free sausages

1 tbsp olive oil

1 onion, chopped

500ml chicken stock, fresh or made with 1 stock cube

Few drops of Worcestershire sauce

2 bay leaves

1 tsp English mustard

2 tsp cornflour, dissolved in a little water

1 x 400g tin butterbeans, rinsed and drained

1 tsp olive oil

Salt and freshly ground black pepper

Boil or steam the potatoes until just tender. Allow to cool completely before cutting into thin slices. Preheat the oven to 160°C/140°C fan/325°F/gas mark 3.

Use kitchen scissors to snip each sausage into three or four pieces. Heat the oil in a large frying pan. Fry the sausages until brown on all sides and then set aside. Reduce the heat to low, add the onion and fry for 5 minutes until softened. Stir in the chicken stock and bring up to a gentle simmer, then add the Worcestershire sauce, bay leaves and mustard. Add the cornflour and stir to thicken.

Arrange the sausages and butterbeans over the base of a large, lidded casserole dish and pour over the sauce. Place one layer of the sliced potatoes over the top of the dish and press lightly into the sauce. Arrange the rest of the potatoes over the top. Drizzle with olive oil and season with salt and pepper.

Place the lid on the casserole dish and cook in the oven for 1 hour. Remove the lid from the dish, increase the oven temperature to 220°C / 200°C fan / 425°F / gas mark 7 and cook for a further 15 minutes until the potatoes are browned.

Vegetarian chilli

Satisfying and filling chilli that's suitable for vegetarians and meat-eaters alike. Serve with a small portion of brown rice or go wild and try it with corn tortillas and soured cream.

SERVES 6   10 mins   1 hour

184 calories

Good carbs ✓

- **800g butternut squash (1 medium), peeled, seeded and cut into 2.5-cm chunks**
- **½ tsp cinnamon**
- **1 tbsp plus 1 tsp olive oil**
- **1 onion, chopped**
- **1 green pepper, seeded and chopped**
- **2 fresh red or green chillies, seeded and sliced into rings**
- **2 cloves garlic, finely chopped**
- **Zest and juice of 1 lime**
- **2 tsp mild chilli powder**
- **2 tsp ground cumin**
- **1 tsp paprika**
- **1 tsp cocoa powder**
- **2 x 400g tins chopped tomatoes**

2 x 400g tins kidney beans, rinsed and drained
Salt and freshly ground black pepper

Preheat the oven to 220°C/200°C fan/425°F/gas mark 7.

Place the butternut squash on a baking tray, sprinkle over the cinnamon and season generously with salt and pepper. Drizzle over 1 tablespoon of olive oil and toss through with your hands. Bake in the oven for 15-20 minutes, until just tender.

Meanwhile, heat the remaining teaspoon of olive oil in a large pan and add the onion, green pepper and chillies. Fry gently for 5 minutes. Add the garlic and lime zest and cook for a further minute or two. Add the cumin, paprika and cocoa powder. Stir through before adding the chopped tomatoes and kidney beans.

Bring up to a gentle simmer and cook, lid off, for about 30 minutes. Add the butternut squash and lime juice and stir through gently. Taste and adjust the seasoning and cook for a further 5 minutes before serving.

The chilli keeps well in the fridge or can be made in advance and frozen.

Chicken casserole

Lovely, hearty comfort food. The great thing about this recipe is that you don't add the chicken until near the end of the cooking time, ensuring that it is beautifully tender. The sauce can be made in advance and frozen before the chicken is added.

SERVES 4   15 mins   2½ hours   **266** calories

Protein-rich ✓

4 slices streaky bacon, roughly chopped
1 onion, chopped
1 carrot, peeled and diced
1 parsnip, peeled and diced
4 small leeks, washed and sliced
1 red pepper, seeded and chopped
250g chestnut mushrooms, washed and sliced
200ml dry white wine
500ml chicken stock, fresh or made with a stock cube
2 bay leaves
400g chicken breast, cut into 2.5-cm dice
Salt and freshly ground black pepper

Preheat the oven to 170°C/150°C fan/325°F/gas mark 3.

Place a large, lidded frying pan or ovenproof casserole over a medium/high heat. When hot add the streaky bacon and fry for 2–3 minutes until just turning brown. Remove the bacon using a slotted spoon and set aside.

Add the onion to the pan and immediately reduce the heat. Leave the onion to cook slowly in the bacon fat for about 5 minutes.

Add the carrot, parsnip, leeks and red pepper to the pan. Stir thoroughly and season with salt and pepper. Turn the heat up a little and continue to cook for a further 3 minutes.

Stir through the mushrooms and add the wine, chicken stock and bay leaves. Bring to a gentle simmer and then transfer to a casserole dish if necessary. Cover and place in the preheated oven and cook for approximately 2 hours. You could also cook this dish in a slow cooker for 6-8 hours.

When you are almost ready to eat, remove from the oven, place over a low/medium heat on the hob and bring up to a gentle simmer. If necessary, add a little extra water at this stage. Add the diced chicken and bring back to simmering point. Then cook gently for 12 minutes. Check the chicken is cooked through before serving.

Melanzane parmigiani

This traditional Italian dish is decadent and deliciously cheesy. The tomato sauce is so good that it can be used in a multitude of other dishes.

SERVES 4 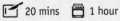 20 mins  1 hour

1 x 400g tin chopped tomatoes
1 x 500g jar tomato passata
3 tbsp olive oil
2 tsp garlic oil
1 heaped tsp soft dark brown sugar
½ tsp mixed Italian herbs
1 tbsp red wine vinegar

600g aubergine (2 large or 3 small)
250g mozzarella
30g Parmesan, grated
Salt and freshly ground black pepper

Place the tomatoes, passata, olive oil and garlic oil in a large, lidded pan. Bring up to a simmer, stirring well so that the oil is incorporated into the sauce.

Reduce the heat to the lowest possible setting and balance the lid on the pan, leaving a small gap for the steam to escape. Cook for 30 minutes, stirring regularly to prevent sticking.

Remove from the heat and stir in the brown sugar, herbs and red wine vinegar. Stir well and season lightly with salt and pepper. Taste and adjust the seasoning, adding a little more salt, vinegar or sugar to get it just right. Leave the sauce to cool completely.

Preheat the oven to 200°C/180°C fan/400°F/gas mark 6.

Trim the aubergine and cut into thin slices, about 4–5mm thick. Cut the mozzarella into thin slices too. Start layering up the melanzane as you would with a lasagne. Take a medium-sized ovenproof dish and put a thin layer of tomato sauce on the bottom. Then add a layer of aubergine, a layer of tomato sauce and finally a layer of mozzarella. Repeat twice more, finishing with a layer of mozzarella. Sprinkle the Parmesan generously over the top.

Bake in the oven for 30 minutes or until the top is bubbling and brown. Leave to stand for 5 minutes before serving.

Chicken korma

This coconutty korma is a brilliant family recipe. You can make and freeze the sauce in advance and just cook the chicken when you're ready to serve. Serve with brown basmati rice.

SERVES 4   40 mins (including marinating time)   40 mins   **428** calories

Healthy fats	✓
Protein-rich	✓

500g skinless chicken breast, diced

2 tbsp natural yoghurt

1 onion

2 cloves garlic

1 large thumb-sized piece of ginger, peeled

1 tbsp rice bran oil

4 cardamom pods, crushed

1 tsp ground cumin

1 tsp ground coriander

½ tsp ground turmeric

½ tsp mild chilli powder

2 cloves, stalks removed

1 bay leaf

30g ground almonds

1 heaped tbsp sugar-free apricot jam

1 x 400g tin coconut milk

Salt and freshly ground black pepper

Toss the chicken in the yoghurt until thoroughly coated. Cover, refrigerate and leave to marinate for at least 30 minutes while you prepare the rest of the dish.

Very finely chop the onion, garlic and ginger. This can be done by hand or in a food processor. Heat the oil gently in a large, lidded non-stick pan. Add the onions, garlic and ginger and stir. Cover and cook slowly, stirring occasionally, for 10–15 minutes until very soft.

Stir in the all the spices and bay leaf and season generously with salt and pepper. Add the almonds, then cook gently with the lid off for 5 minutes, stirring frequently.

Scoop about 2 tablespoons of the cream off the top of the tin of coconut milk and stir into the sauce until simmering. Stir in the apricot jam and then add a little of the thin coconut water. Reserve the remaining liquid to add to the sauce later if it is too thick. Simmer, uncovered, for 10 minutes. The sauce can now be used straight away or chilled or frozen for later use.

Bring the sauce to a simmer and add the marinated chicken pieces. Cook for 10–12 minutes until cooked through and tender (the time will vary depending on the size of the chicken pieces).

Classic bolognaise

This is another family favourite that I cook in bulk and freeze in suitable portions. I like to slow cook this overnight but 2 hours at 160°C/140°C fan/325°F/gas mark 3 would work just as well. Don't be put off by the long list of ingredients, this is really a 'bung-it-in-the-pan-and-forget-about-it' recipe.

SERVES 8   15 mins   2½ hours   **299** calories

Protein-rich ✓

1 tbsp olive oil

1 large onion, diced

½ tsp salt

1kg lean minced beef

2 cloves garlic, sliced

1 red pepper, seeded and diced

1 green pepper, seeded and diced

1 courgette, peeled and diced

2 x 400g tins whole tomatoes

2 tbsp tomato purée

250g mushrooms, washed and sliced

Generous splash of Worcestershire sauce

1 tsp mushroom ketchup (or soy sauce)

1 tbsp red wine vinegar

2 bay leaves

1 tsp dried mixed Italian herbs

200ml red wine

Freshly ground black pepper

Heat the oil in a very large flameproof casserole over a medium heat. Add the onion and salt to the pan and fry for 5 minutes.

Break up the mince with your hands and add to the pan. Turn the heat up a little and fry, stirring very frequently, until all the meat is broken up and no pink remains.

Add the chopped peppers and courgette and stir in. Add the tinned tomatoes, breaking them up a little with your spoon as you do so. Add the tomato purée, mushrooms, Worcestershire sauce, mushroom ketchup, red wine vinegar, bay leaves, dried herbs and season with black pepper.

Bring up to a simmer and cook on the hob, uncovered, for about 30 minutes. Add the red wine and either transfer to a slow cooker for about 8 hours or put the lid on the pan and cook in an oven preheated to 160°C/140°C fan/325°F/gas mark 3 for 2 hours.

Lasagne with courgette pasta

Once you have a batch of bolognaise sauce made up, putting together this delicious lasagne is a breeze.

SERVES 4   1¼ hours (including salting time)   30 mins   **336** calories

Protein-rich ✓

1 large courgette, washed
300ml milk
30g butter
1 tbsp cornflour, dissolved in a little water
30g cream cheese
50g Cheddar, grated
30g Parmesan, finely grated
500g Classic Bolognaise (page 183)
Salt and freshly ground black pepper

Trim the ends off the courgette. Use a vegetable peeler to peel fat ribbons of courgette. Discard the first piece, which is mainly skin and keep making slivers until you reach the seeds in the middle. Turn the courgette over and do the same on the other side. Place the slices in a colander and scatter generously with salt. Leave to drain for 1 hour. Rinse away the salt and dry on kitchen paper before using.

Place the milk and butter in non-stick pan and bring to a simmer. Add the cornflour paste a little at a time, stirring continuously. Remove from the heat and season with salt and pepper. Stir in the cream cheese and then add the Cheddar and Parmesan, reserving a small quantity of each for the top of the lasagne.

Preheat the oven to 190°C/170°C fan/375°F/gas mark 5.

In a large ovenproof dish, start assembling the lasagne. Begin with a generous layer of bolognaise sauce, then a single layer of courgette, then a small amount of cheese sauce. Continue layering bolognaise, courgette and cheese sauce, ending with a thick layer of cheese sauce.

Sprinkle over the reserved Cheddar and Parmesan and then bake in the oven for 30 minutes, until browned and bubbling.

Smoky pork 'chilli'

This versatile family favourite is one of the most popular dishes round our house. I often make double quantities of this recipe and freeze in batches.

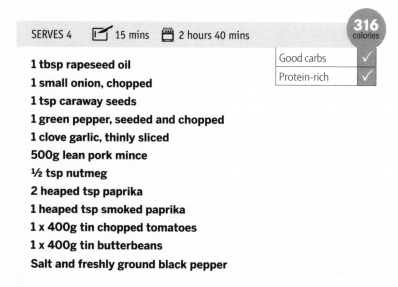

SERVES 4   15 mins   2 hours 40 mins   **316** calories

| Good carbs | ✓ |
| Protein-rich | ✓ |

1 tbsp rapeseed oil
1 small onion, chopped
1 tsp caraway seeds
1 green pepper, seeded and chopped
1 clove garlic, thinly sliced
500g lean pork mince
½ tsp nutmeg
2 heaped tsp paprika
1 heaped tsp smoked paprika
1 x 400g tin chopped tomatoes
1 x 400g tin butterbeans
Salt and freshly ground black pepper

Heat the oil in a large pan or casserole dish. Toss in the onion and caraway seeds. Fry lightly for 5 minutes before adding the green pepper and garlic. Cook for a further 2 minutes.

Break up the mince with your hands and drop it into the pan. Sprinkle over the rest of the spices and season generously with salt and pepper. Turn the heat up and stir continuously until the meat is cooked through.

Add the tinned tomatoes and the butterbeans with half of their liquid. Bring up to simmering point and cook, lid off, for approximately 30 minutes. Meanwhile, preheat the oven to 160°C/140°C fan/325°F/gas mark 3.

Transfer the chilli to an ovenproof dish if necessary and cover the dish with a lid or foil. Cook in the oven for a further 2 hours. Alternatively, transfer to a slow cooker and cook for 6–8 hours.

Serve with brown rice or a jacket potato and some green vegetables on the side.

Tabbouleh parsley salad

This Middle Eastern salad is fresh and interesting. It's traditionally made with bulgur wheat but I make it here with quinoa. To turn this into a full meal you could simply stir in some cooked jumbo prawns or some cheese such as Wensleydale. But my absolute favourite way to eat this is with Mini Falafel Burgers (page 188), a generous dollop of good houmous and a few olives. Yum yum yum.

107 calories

SERVES 2   10 mins, plus quinoa cooking time

20g quinoa or 50g cooked quinoa
200g tomatoes
2 spring onions
Juice of 1 lemon
¼ tsp ground cinnamon
¼ tsp ground coriander
Pinch of ground nutmeg
Pinch of ground cloves
Pinch of ground ginger
50g fresh flat-leaf parsley
1 tbsp mild olive oil
Salt and freshly ground black pepper

Healthy fats	✓
Good carbs	✓

Cook the quinoa according to the instructions on the packet and place in a bowl.

Finely chop the tomatoes and spring onions and add to the quinoa. Squeeze in the lemon juice and season generously with salt and pepper. Stir, add all the spices and stir again.

Chop the parsley very finely, discarding any thick stems. Stir into the salad with the olive oil. Leave to rest for 5 minutes before serving.

Mini falafel burgers

Falafels are a quick, easy fix for dinner with the family. I can throw them together and have them on the table in 10 minutes, perfect with a simple salad of rocket, cherry tomatoes and sliced red onion. If you have any left over you can keep them in the fridge – they're great in a lunch box the following day. Chickpeas are such a star ingredient – delicious and versatile with a very healthy balance of good carbohydrates, fibre and protein.

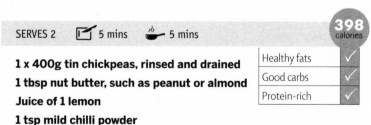

SERVES 2	5 mins	5 mins	**398** calories

1 x 400g tin chickpeas, rinsed and drained

1 tbsp nut butter, such as peanut or almond

Juice of 1 lemon

1 tsp mild chilli powder

1 tsp ground cumin

1 tbsp gram (chickpea) flour

2 tbsp rice bran oil

Healthy fats	✓
Good carbs	✓
Protein-rich	✓

Salt and freshly ground black pepper
Wedge of lemon, to serve

Place the chickpeas in a food processor with the nut butter, lemon juice, chilli powder, ground cumin and gram flour. Season generously with salt and pepper. Whizz until nearly smooth and well combined – you want to leave a few bigger bits of chickpea for a more interesting texture.

Use a teaspoon to take out heaps of the mixture and place on a chopping board. Use the back of a spoon to flatten each heap slightly.

Heat the oil in a wide frying pan over a medium heat. When hot, carefully arrange the falafels in the pan. Cook for 2–3 minutes until a beautiful golden brown on the underside. Turn the falafels over carefully and press into the pan with a spatula. Cook for a further 2–3 minutes until cooked through and golden all over. Remove from the pan and drain on kitchen paper to absorb off excess oil before serving. Serve hot or cold with a wedge of lemon to squeeze over.

Sides and Veggies

Rice dishes

Rice is an important part of eating well, yet it can be considered dull and boring. One of my favourite ways to make rice an important and integral part of the meal is to combine it with new flavours and lots of vegetables.

All the rice recipes I've included here use cooked rice (basmati or brown), so I would either cook the rice in advance or use a pre-cooked pouch. A 30g portion of dry rice translates to an 80g portion of cooked rice and this is the portion size you should be looking for. Frequently I use a pouch of rice that contains 250g cooked rice. This makes enough rice for 3 servings, so that's a meal for two in the evening, followed by a tupperware of cold rice for lunch the next day. Once the rice is cooked, all of these dishes take less than 10 minutes to prepare.

Big Indian green rice

This rice goes well with any curry or with red meats such as lamb or pork.

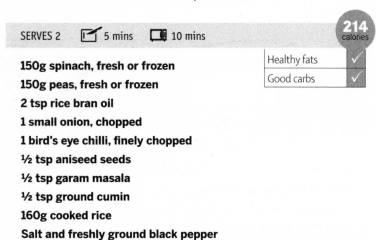

SERVES 2   5 mins   10 mins   **214** calories

150g spinach, fresh or frozen

150g peas, fresh or frozen

2 tsp rice bran oil

1 small onion, chopped

1 bird's eye chilli, finely chopped

½ tsp aniseed seeds

½ tsp garam masala

½ tsp ground cumin

160g cooked rice

Salt and freshly ground black pepper

Healthy fats	✓
Good carbs	✓

Place the spinach and peas in a microwave-safe bowl and cover with cling film, leaving a 2cm gap at the side for steam to escape. Cook for about 3 minutes if using fresh or 5 minutes from frozen. Set aside to cool.

Heat the oil in a heavy-based wide pan over a high heat. Add the onion, chilli and aniseed seeds. Cook 2 minutes over a high heat then reduce the heat and cook for another 5 minutes, until the onions are soft and translucent.

Add the garam masala and cumin and stir through. Add the spinach, peas and rice and stir well until warmed through. Season with salt and pepper and serve.

Sweet Indian red rice

This rice goes well with chicken or prawn dishes simply stirring cooked chicken or prawns into the rice will create a quick and easy dinner.

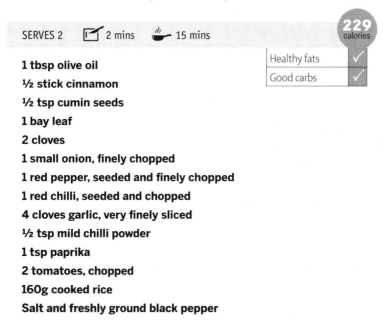

SERVES 2   2 mins   15 mins   **229** calories

| Healthy fats | ✓ |
| Good carbs | ✓ |

1 tbsp olive oil
½ stick cinnamon
½ tsp cumin seeds
1 bay leaf
2 cloves
1 small onion, finely chopped
1 red pepper, seeded and finely chopped
1 red chilli, seeded and chopped
4 cloves garlic, very finely sliced
½ tsp mild chilli powder
1 tsp paprika
2 tomatoes, chopped
160g cooked rice
Salt and freshly ground black pepper

Heat the oil in a heavy-based wide pan. Add the cinnamon, cumin seeds, bay leaf and cloves. Fry for 1 minute, or until they just start to release their aroma. Add the onion, red pepper and chilli and fry over a medium/high heat for 5 minutes.

Add the garlic, chilli powder, paprika and tomatoes and reduce the heat. Season generously with salt and pepper and cook for another 5–7 minutes.

Remove the cinnamon stick, bay leaf and cloves and then add the cooked rice and mix well. Warm the rice through for a few minutes before serving.

Mediterranean rice

This versatile rice will jazz up many meat or chicken dishes. Serve simply with a pork chop or some grilled chicken for a quick and tasty meal.

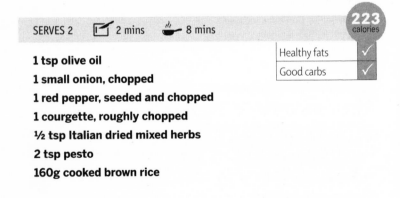

SERVES 2   2 mins   8 mins   **223** calories

| Healthy fats | ✓ |
| Good carbs | ✓ |

1 tsp olive oil
1 small onion, chopped
1 red pepper, seeded and chopped
1 courgette, roughly chopped
½ tsp Italian dried mixed herbs
2 tsp pesto
160g cooked brown rice

Heat the olive oil in a pan over a medium heat and gently fry the onion, red pepper and courgette for a few minutes, until tender.

Stir through the mixed herbs and pesto.

Add the rice and continue to cook over a low/medium heat until warmed through.

Sticky coconut rice

This Thai rice makes a great side dish but is so moreish that I often eat it on it's own, sometimes adding a handful of cooked prawns to make a more complete meal.

SERVES 2   2 mins   8 mins   **386** calories

Good carbs ✓

1 tsp olive oil
200g pak choi, trimmed and washed
200g mushrooms, washed and sliced
1 tsp walnut oil
1 tbsp fish sauce
Zest of 1 lime
½ x 400g tin coconut milk
160g cooked brown rice
Juice of ½ lime

Heat the olive oil in a wide, deep frying pan. Cut the leaves off the pak choi and save for later. Dice the thick stems of the pak choi and add to the pan. Fry for a minute or two before adding the mushrooms. Cook over a high heat until tender, about 3 minutes. Stir through the walnut oil, fish sauce and the lime zest.

Roughly chop the pak choi leaves and add to the pan. From the tin of coconut milk, add about 2 tablespoons of the thick creamy bit from the top and one tablespoon of the coconut water from the bottom. Stir in and cook until bubbling.

Add the rice and simmer until the liquid has nearly evaporated. Remove from the heat and stir through the lime juice.

Three pepper pilau rice

This distinctive yellow rice has a subtle flavour that complements both Asian and British dishes.

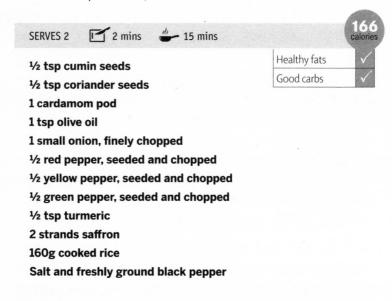

SERVES 2   2 mins   15 mins

166 calories

½ tsp cumin seeds
½ tsp coriander seeds
1 cardamom pod
1 tsp olive oil
1 small onion, finely chopped
½ red pepper, seeded and chopped
½ yellow pepper, seeded and chopped
½ green pepper, seeded and chopped
½ tsp turmeric
2 strands saffron
160g cooked rice
Salt and freshly ground black pepper

| Healthy fats | ✓ |
| Good carbs | ✓ |

Crush the cumin seeds, coriander seeds and cardamom pod in a pestle and mortar. Heat a heavy-based frying pan over a high heat and dry fry these spices for 1 minute.

Turn the heat right down and add the oil, chopped onion and peppers. Fry slowly until soft and translucent, about 10 minutes.

Add the rest of the spices, salt and pepper and stir through.

Add the cooked rice and stir well until warmed through.

Roasted butternut squash

Compared to potatoes or sweet potatoes, butternut squash has less impact on your blood sugar, so makes an excellent accompaniment to meat or chicken dishes.

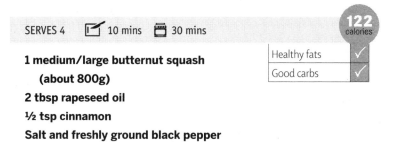

SERVES 4   ☑ 10 mins   🗂 30 mins   **122** calories

**1 medium/large butternut squash
    (about 800g)**
2 tbsp rapeseed oil
½ tsp cinnamon
Salt and freshly ground black pepper

| Healthy fats | ✓ |
| Good carbs | ✓ |

Preheat the oven to 220°C/200°C fan/425°F/gas mark 7.

Using a very sharp knife, top and tail the squash before cutting off the skin. Cut the squash in half lengthways and scoop out the pith and seeds. Cut into rough chunks or slices.

Place the squash in a baking dish and pour over the oil. Season generously with salt and pepper and sprinkle over the cinnamon. Use your hands to toss the oil through the squash, making sure it is all evenly covered.

Bake in the oven for 20–30 minutes, until tender.

Balsamic glaze and dressing

Make either a beautiful glaze for meat and salads or turn it into a complete dressing. Keep in a small glass bottle (I use a mini wine bottle) and place proudly on the table. You'll find many, many uses for this glaze.

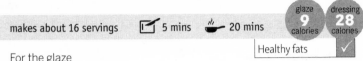

makes about 16 servings   5 mins   20 mins   glaze **9** calories   dressing **28** calories

Healthy fats ✓

For the glaze
100ml light balsamic vinegar
1 heaped tsp set honey

For the dressing
50ml extra-virgin olive oil
Juice of half lemon
Salt and freshly ground black pepper

To make the glaze, simply heat the balsamic vinegar and honey together in a small non-stick pan. Bring to a very gentle simmer and cook over a low heat for about 20 minutes or until the mixture sticks to the back of a spoon. Allow to cool in the pan before transferring to a bottle or using to make a balsamic dressing.

To make the dressing, whisk together the balsamic glaze with the rest of the ingredients. Transfer to a bottle or jar and the dressing will keep for several weeks.

Tomato ketchup

Make your own tomato ketchup using this simple recipe. It's far healthier than the shop-bought version. I keep it in a fancy bottle in the fridge so that my children get that authentic ketchup feeling.

SERVES 12   2 mins   25 mins   **8** calories

50g tomato pureé
1 tsp onion salt
150g passata
30ml red wine vinegar
¼ tsp garlic purée

Heat the tomato purée in a non-stick pan over a medium heat for 2 minutes, stirring continuously. This makes the purée sweeter.

Add the rest of the ingredients and stir well. Place a lid on the pan, leaving a gap at one side for steam to escape. Bring to a simmer and cook for about 20 minutes, stirring every few minutes, or until a thick consistency is reached.

Transfer to a bottle or jar and it will keep in the fridge for up to 2 weeks.

Variation

Hot and smoky sauce

Add a few drops of Worcestershire sauce, ½ teaspoon of mild chilli powder, a few drops of Tabasco and ½ teaspoon of smoked paprika for a more 'grown up' ketchup.

Chilli and lime dip

This is an easy-to-put-together sauce that adds pizzazz to a summery lunch or barbecue.

SERVES 4   2 mins

23 calories

2 tbsp French-style mayonnaise
1 tsp chilli flakes
Pinch of salt
Juice of 1 lime
Small handful of fresh coriander, finely chopped

Simply mix all the ingredients together in a small bowl until well combined and leave for a few minutes for the flavours to infuse.

Caribbean barbecue sauce

This sticky sauce enhances the flavour of meat, especially chicken. Rub on to the meat just before cooking or coat cooked meat in a generous portion of sauce as you serve.

SERVES 6   2 mins

26 calories

2 tsp soft dark brown sugar
½ tsp smoked paprika
1 tsp dried oregano
2 tsp cornflour
2 tsp Dijon mustard
1 tsp maple syrup

½ tsp Worcestershire sauce

2 tsp cider vinegar

1 tsp black treacle

1 tsp onion salt

Simply whisk all the ingredients together in a small bowl. If it's too thick add a little water so it is just pourable. Transfer to a lidded jar and keep in the fridge until needed.

Tzatziki

This yoghurt sauce goes well with sticks of raw vegetables for snacking, with veggie burgers as an alternative to ketchup, or with Indian food.

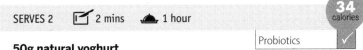

SERVES 2   2 mins   1 hour   **34** calories

Probiotics ✓

50g natural yoghurt

2.5cm piece of cucumber, unpeeled and grated

1 tsp fresh lemon juice

½ tsp extra-virgin olive oil

1 fresh basil leaf, finely chopped

Pinch of salt

Simply mix all the ingredients together and leave the flavours to develop for about an hour before serving.

Cajun spice rub

By just mixing together this simple collection of spices you can make an incredibly delicious rub that works well on almost any meat or fish. I use it on chicken and salmon before baking in the oven and on anything that goes on the barbecue.

SERVES 12   🕐 2 mins

5 tsp ground cumin
2 heaped tsp smoked paprika
2 heaped tsp hot paprika
2 tsp dried thyme
2 tsp dried oregano
½ tsp cayenne pepper
1 tsp salt

Place all the ingredients into a small, lidded jar. I recycle an old spice jar for this – but remember to re-label it! Give it a very good shake. The spice mix will keep for up to a month.

Sprinkle about a teaspoon on to meat or fish with a drizzle of oil. Rub all over the meat and leave to rest for 5 minutes before cooking.

Salsa in a jar

I'm a big fan of a salsa dip. It's not high in calories and home-made is always better than shop-bought. This recipe will make 2–4 jars. It will keep for months sealed in an airtight container or for a couple of weeks in the fridge once opened.

SERVES 16  4 mins  5 mins

1 small onion, finely diced
½ green pepper, seeded and finely diced
2 x 400g tins chopped tomatoes (whizz in a food processor if you prefer a smooth-textured salsa)
2 tbsp tomato purée
30g green jalapeños (from a jar, drained weight), finely chopped
½ clove garlic, finely chopped
Juice of 1 lime
1 tbsp red wine vinegar
Pinch of salt
Handful of fresh coriander, finely chopped (optional)
¼ tsp ground cumin
¼ tsp mild chilli powder

Place the chopped onion and green pepper in a microwave-safe bowl, add a tablespoon of water and cover with cling film. Make a small slit in the cling film to allow steam to escape. Cook on high for 3–4 minutes until soft.

Now simply place everything in a large bowl and stir thoroughly. Taste and adjust the seasoning before transferring to clean jars. You can recycle old jars for this, just check that they have the plastic coating inside the lids – this is white rather than metal and is needed to stop the metal being corroded by the vinegar. You can sterilise the jars and lids in the top shelf of a dishwasher.

For best results, allow the flavours of the salsa to develop for 24 hours before eating.

Puddings

Classic vanilla ice cream

There is no need for an ice cream maker with this recipe.
Remove from the freezer about 10 minutes before serving.

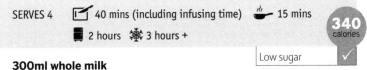

SERVES 4   40 mins (including infusing time)   15 mins

2 hours   3 hours +

340 calories

Low sugar ✓

300ml whole milk
30g stevia
1 vanilla pod
3 large egg yolks
30g caster sugar
1 tsp granulated sugar
300ml double cream

Pour the milk into a pan and add the stevia. Slit the vanilla pod in half lengthways and scrape out as many seeds as you can into the milk. Cut the pod into quarters and add it to the pan. Heat the milk until just simmering, then take it off the heat and leave for 30 minutes for the flavours to infuse. Remove and discard the vanilla pod pieces.

Put the egg yolks into a clean bowl with the caster sugar. Beat the egg yolks for about 2 minutes until thick and pale. Beat about 100ml of the vanilla milk into the egg yolks, one tablespoon at a time.

Reheat the rest of the milk until just simmering, then take off the heat and stir in the egg yolk mixture. Return the pan to a very low heat and cook, stirring continuously, until thickened; this will take about 10 minutes. Do not allow it to boil. As soon as it coats the back of a spoon, remove from the heat and pour into a heatproof bowl or jug. Sprinkle on the granulated sugar to stop a skin forming. When it has cooled sufficiently, transfer to the fridge and leave to chill thoroughly.

Whip the cream in a large bowl until light and floppy but not too stiff. Fold it into the cold custard. Transfer to a freezer container and freeze for 3 hours, mixing with a fork every hour to stop ice crystals forming.

Black cherry yoghurt

If you are missing processed fruit yoghurts then this is a simple and delicious way to make your own. Black cherry is my favourite yoghurt flavour but you can use the same technique with any red berries or soft fruit such as peaches and apricots.

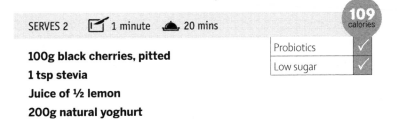

SERVES 2   1 minute   20 mins   **109** calories

| Probiotics | ✓ |
| Low sugar | ✓ |

100g black cherries, pitted
1 tsp stevia
Juice of ½ lemon
200g natural yoghurt

Roughly chop the cherries and place in a small bowl with the stevia and lemon juice. Stir and leave to rest for 20 minutes for the flavours to ooze out of the fruit.

Stir in the natural yoghurt and divide between two bowls.

Crustless strawberry and custard tartlets

I have used a small quantity of light brown sugar in this recipe, but feel free to change this to a combination of sugar and sweetener.

SERVES 4    5 mins   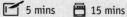 15 mins   **308** calories

Butter for greasing
100g fresh strawberries, washed, hulled and thickly sliced
1 large egg
2 large egg yolks
50g soft light brown sugar
150ml double cream
50g natural yoghurt
Juice of ½ lemon

Preheat the oven to 170°C/150°C fan/325°F/gas mark 3. Line the base of 4 individual tart tins with a circle of baking parchment and lightly grease the sides. Alternatively you can use ramekins and serve the dessert in the dish.

Place the tart tins on a baking tray. Arrange the strawberries equally between the 4 tins.

Whisk the egg and egg yolks together in a jug. Add the sugar and whisk again before stirring in the cream, yoghurt and finally the lemon juice. Pour the mixture over the strawberries in the tart tins, giving each tin a little shake so that the mixture is distributed evenly.

Place the baking tray in the oven and bake for 12–15 minutes, until the filling is just firm.

Individual pistachio ice creams

*Decadent and easy, these ice creams are poured into disposable
plastic cups before being frozen. To serve, run the cup under
the hot tap before turning upside down on to a plate.*

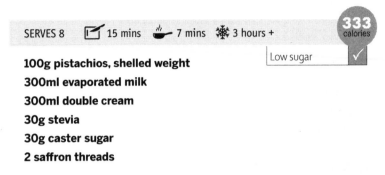

SERVES 8   15 mins   7 mins   3 hours +   **333** calories

Low sugar ✓

100g pistachios, shelled weight
300ml evaporated milk
300ml double cream
30g stevia
30g caster sugar
2 saffron threads

Reserve a small handful of pistachios to serve and place the rest
of the pistachios in a food processor and chop until finely ground.

Place the evaporated milk, cream, stevia and caster sugar in a
non-stick pan and bring to simmering point, stirring frequently to
stop it catching on the bottom of the pan.

When it starts to bubble, stir in the ground pistachios and
saffron. Continue to bubble gently for a further 5 minutes.

Leave to cool in the pan then transfer to a jug and refrigerate
until chilled. Divide the cream equally between 8 plastic cups,
cover with cling film and freeze.

Upturn the pistachio ice creams onto plates. Roughly chop the
remaining pistachios and sprinkle over the top.

Microwave chocolate pudding

Yes, this pudding IS as good as it sounds.

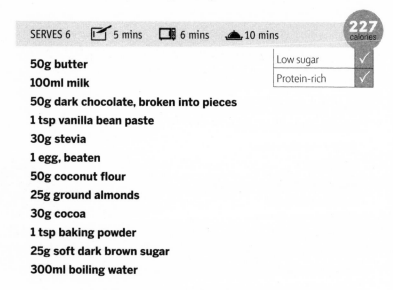

SERVES 6   5 mins   6 mins   10 mins   **227** calories

50g butter

100ml milk

50g dark chocolate, broken into pieces

1 tsp vanilla bean paste

30g stevia

1 egg, beaten

50g coconut flour

25g ground almonds

30g cocoa

1 tsp baking powder

25g soft dark brown sugar

300ml boiling water

Low sugar	✓
Protein-rich	✓

Place the butter, milk and dark chocolate in a large microwave-safe bowl. Pulse in the microwave for 30-second intervals until the chocolate and butter have completely melted into the milk.

Stir in the vanilla, stevia and beaten egg, making sure the stevia is fully dissolved.

In a separate bowl mix the coconut flour, ground almonds, half the cocoa and the baking powder. Pour the dry ingredients into the milk and chocolate mixture and stir until all the lumps are gone.

Mix the remaining cocoa with the dark brown sugar and sprinkle over the top. Gently pour the boiling water over the top of the pudding.

Place in the microwave with a plate over the top. Cook for 6 minutes on high (in an 800W microwave). Leave to rest for 10 minutes with the plate still on. Serve directly from the bowl.

Crushed berry frozen yoghurt

This is a great staple to have on standby in the freezer. Don't forget to get it out of the freezer 10–15 minutes before serving.

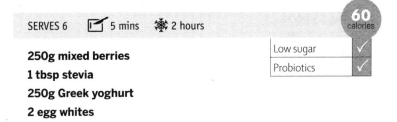

| SERVES 6 | 5 mins | 2 hours | | **60** calories |

250g mixed berries
1 tbsp stevia
250g Greek yoghurt
2 egg whites

| Low sugar | ✓ |
| Probiotics | ✓ |

Place the mixed berries in a large bowl and crush well until you have lots of juice, but still some chunks of fruit remaining. Stir in the stevia and then the Greek yoghurt.

Place the egg whites in a separate bowl and whisk until they form stiff peaks. Fold into the berries and yoghurt mixture.

Transfer to a freezer container and freeze for 2 hours. Remove from the freezer and stir the mixture thoroughly using a fork to break up any ice crystals. Return to the freezer where it can be stored for up to 3 months.

Baked pears with blue cheese

Somewhere between a dessert and a cheese course, this dish has sophistication written all over it.

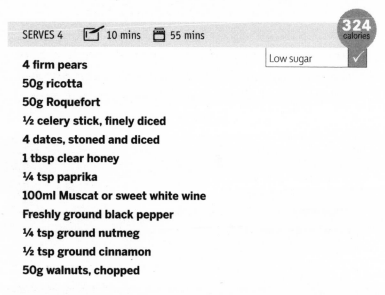

SERVES 4   10 mins   55 mins

324 calories

Low sugar ✓

4 firm pears
50g ricotta
50g Roquefort
½ celery stick, finely diced
4 dates, stoned and diced
1 tbsp clear honey
¼ tsp paprika
100ml Muscat or sweet white wine
Freshly ground black pepper
¼ tsp ground nutmeg
½ tsp ground cinnamon
50g walnuts, chopped

Preheat the oven to 160°C/140°C fan/325°F/gas mark 3.

Cut the pears in half lengthways. Use a teaspoon or sharp knife to cut out the seeds and core in the centre of each pear half. Arrange the pears, cut side up, in a baking dish.

In a small bowl, combine the ricotta, Roquefort, celery, dates, honey and paprika. Put a heaped teaspoon of the mix into the centre of each pear. Pour the sweet wine around the pears and then season with black pepper, nutmeg and cinnamon. Cover with foil and bake in the oven for 45 minutes, or until just tender.

Increase the heat to 190°C/170°C fan/375°F/gas mark 5. Remove the foil from the dish and sprinkle over the chopped walnuts before returning to the oven, uncovered, for a further 10 minutes.

Dark chocolate mousse

These extreme chocolate mousses don't really need any added sugar. But if you find you need a little extra sweetness then add 2 teaspoons of stevia or a tablespoon of sugar to the melted chocolate.

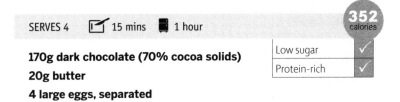

SERVES 4   15 mins   1 hour   **352** calories

170g dark chocolate (70% cocoa solids)
20g butter
4 large eggs, separated

| Low sugar | ✓ |
| Protein-rich | ✓ |

Place a small heatproof bowl over a pan of gently simmering water, making sure the base of the bowl does not touch the water. Break the chocolate into small pieces and add to the bowl along with the butter. Heat until it melts and then remove from the heat.

Beat the egg yolks gently and then pour into the melted chocolate. Stir until well combined.

Whisk the egg whites until they form stiff peaks. Add a third of the egg whites to the melted chocolate and mix well. Then fold in the rest of the egg whites very gently, trying not to knock too much air out of the whites. Divide the mousse between 4 small serving dishes and chill for at least an hour before serving.

Summer fruit pudding

A great summer favourite, this pudding can be made with practically any combination of berries – fresh or frozen.

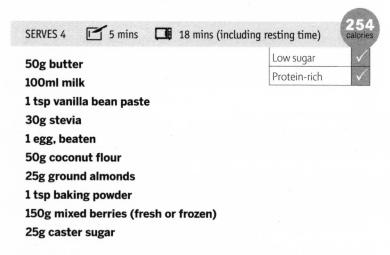

SERVES 4 | 5 mins | 18 mins (including resting time) | **254** calories

Low sugar	✓
Protein-rich	✓

50g butter
100ml milk
1 tsp vanilla bean paste
30g stevia
1 egg, beaten
50g coconut flour
25g ground almonds
1 tsp baking powder
150g mixed berries (fresh or frozen)
25g caster sugar

Place the butter and milk in a microwave-safe bowl. Heat in the microwave for 30-second blasts until the butter has completely melted into the milk. Do not let the milk boil. Stir in the vanilla, stevia and beaten egg, making sure the stevia is fully dissolved.

In a separate bowl mix the coconut flour, ground almonds and baking powder. Pour in the sweetened milk mixture and stir well.

Lightly butter a large microwave-safe bowl. Place the berries in the bottom of the bowl and spoon the pudding mixture over the top. Sprinkle the caster sugar over the top.

Place in the microwave with a plate over the top. If you are using fresh berries cook for 6 minutes (800W microwave); if frozen cook for 8 minutes. Leave to rest for 10 minutes, still covered by the plate. Turn the bowl upside down on to a clean plate and allow the pudding to sink down on to the plate. Serve warm.

Lemon posset

This cheery lemon mousse tastes divine.

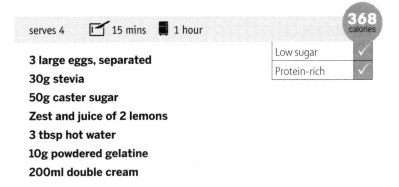

serves 4   15 mins   1 hour

368 calories

3 large eggs, separated
30g stevia
50g caster sugar
Zest and juice of 2 lemons
3 tbsp hot water
10g powdered gelatine
200ml double cream

| Low sugar | ✓ |
| Protein-rich | ✓ |

Place the egg yolks, stevia, caster sugar, lemon zest and juice in a bowl and whisk together with an electric whisk until the sugar has dissolved and the mixture is starting to thicken.

Place the hot water in a small bowl or jug and sprinkle over the gelatine. Stir briskly until thoroughly mixed.

In a separate bowl, whip the cream until it forms soft peaks, then stir in the gelatine. Fold the cream into the egg yolk mixture.

With a clean whisk, whisk the egg whites in a separate bowl until soft peaks form. Gently fold the egg whites into the yolk mixture. Transfer to 4 separate bowls or ramekins and place in the fridge for an hour or until set.

Strawberry cheesecake

This is a star pudding in our house. It looks great and the pecan cheesecake base is such a winner.

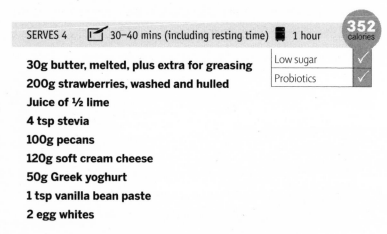

SERVES 4   30–40 mins (including resting time)   1 hour   **352** calories

Low sugar	✓
Probiotics	✓

30g butter, melted, plus extra for greasing
200g strawberries, washed and hulled
Juice of ½ lime
4 tsp stevia
100g pecans
120g soft cream cheese
50g Greek yoghurt
1 tsp vanilla bean paste
2 egg whites

Roughly chop half the strawberries and place them in a bowl with the lime juice and 3 teaspoons of the stevia. Mix and leave to rest for 20–30 minutes.

Lightly grease a small, loose-bottomed cake tin (about 15cm in diameter).

Place the pecans in a food processor and blitz under well ground. Stir into the melted butter and add the remaining teaspoon of stevia. Press the pecan mix into the base of the cake tin, using your fingers to smooth and push the pecans into any gaps. Chill in the fridge while you prepare the topping.

Place the soft cheese in a bowl and mash with a fork. Add the Greek yoghurt and vanilla bean paste and stir until smooth. Add the chopped strawberry mixture including all the lovely pink juice.

In a separate bowl, whisk the egg whites until they form stiff peaks. Stir about a third of the egg whites into the strawberry mixture and then fold in the rest. Scoop the topping over the cheesecake base.

Slice the remaining fresh strawberries and arrange over the top of the cheesecake. Place in the fridge to chill and lightly set before serving.

Individual fluffy apple crumbles

These amazing puddings can be frozen before baking; just cook straight from the freezer and add an extra 10 minutes to the cooking time.

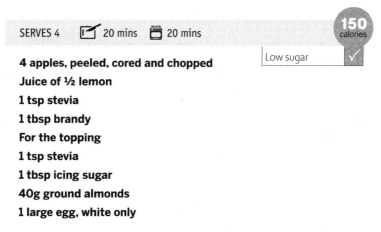

SERVES 4   20 mins   20 mins

150 calories

4 apples, peeled, cored and chopped
Juice of ½ lemon
1 tsp stevia
1 tbsp brandy
For the topping
1 tsp stevia
1 tbsp icing sugar
40g ground almonds
1 large egg, white only

Low sugar ✓

Preheat the oven to 160°C/140°C fan/325°F/gas mark 3.

Put the chopped apples in a lidded pan with the lemon juice, stevia, brandy and 3 tablespoons of water. Bring to the boil and simmer, covered, for 10 minutes. Uncover, turn the heat up and cook for a further 5 minutes until the sauce has thickened. Spoon the apples and sauce into 4 ramekins.

To make the topping, mix the stevia, icing sugar and ground almonds together in a bowl. In a clean bowl, whisk the egg white until it forms stiff peaks, then fold into the dry ingredients. Spoon over the apples and shake gently to level the mixture.

Bake in the oven for 20 minutes.

13

Baking and Cakes

Spiced apple cake

This deliciously fragrant cake is moist and not too sweet.

SERVES 8   🖊 10 mins   🍳 1 hour   **268** calories

Low sugar ✓

75g butter, melted, plus extra for greasing
100g ground almonds
50g coconut flour
30g desiccated coconut
½ tsp baking powder
½ tsp bicarbonate of soda
½ tsp xanthan gum
1½ tsp ground cinnamon
¼ tsp ground nutmeg
1 tbsp caster sugar
1 tbsp stevia
2 large eggs
2 eating apples, peeled and coarsely grated

1 tsp vanilla bean paste
75g natural yoghurt
4 tbsp water

For the topping
2 heaped tbsp soft cream cheese
1 heaped tbsp double cream
1 tsp vanilla bean paste
1 tsp stevia

Preheat the oven to 170°C/150°C fan/325°F/gas mark 3 and lightly grease a small (1lb) loaf tin.

In a large bowl, mix together the ground almonds, coconut flour, desiccated coconut, baking powder, bicarbonate of soda, Xanthan gum, cinnamon, nutmeg and stevia.

In a separate bowl, whisk the eggs with a fork and then stir in the grated apple, melted butter, vanilla, yoghurt and water. Tip the wet ingredients into the dry ingredients and stir well.

Spoon the cake batter into the prepared loaf tin. Level out the batter and bake in the oven for 50–60 minutes, or until a skewer inserted in the centre comes out clean. Transfer to a wire rack and leave to cool completely before icing.

To make the topping, simply mix the cream cheese, cream, vanilla and stevia together and spread over the cake.

Coconut crumbles

These have to be my favourite 'anytime' biscuits. Quick to make with no compromise on taste or texture.

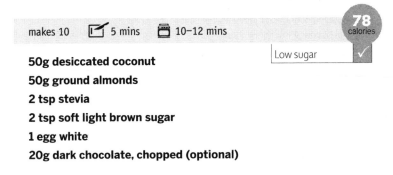

makes 10   5 mins   10–12 mins   **78** calories

Low sugar ✓

50g desiccated coconut
50g ground almonds
2 tsp stevia
2 tsp soft light brown sugar
1 egg white
20g dark chocolate, chopped (optional)

Preheat the oven to 190°C/170°C fan/375°F/gas mark 5 and line a baking tray with baking parchment.

Place the coconut, ground almonds, stevia and sugar in a mixing bowl and stir well.

In a separate bowl, use an electric whisk to beat the egg white until it forms stiff peaks. Stir about a third of the egg white into the coconut mixture and then gently fold in the rest of the egg white until you have a stiff dough.

Take a heaped teaspoon of the mixture and place in the palm of your hand. Place your other hand on top and flatten until you have small thick disc. This mixture will make 8–12 small biscuits, depending on size.

Place the discs on the prepared baking tray and bake in the oven for 10–12 minutes, until gently browned on the edges. Remove to a cooling rack.

When the biscuits have cooled, melt the chocolate gently in

the microwave or in a heatproof bowl set over a pan of gently simmering water. Drizzle the melted chocolate over the crumbles and leave to harden before storing in an airtight container.

Chocolate freezer brittle

This is a great emergency treat to keep in your freezer.

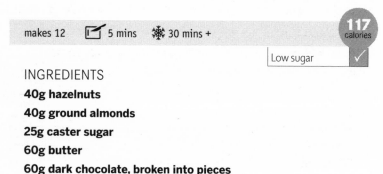

makes 12   5 mins   30 mins +   **117** calories

Low sugar ✓

INGREDIENTS
40g hazelnuts
40g ground almonds
25g caster sugar
60g butter
60g dark chocolate, broken into pieces

Place the hazelnuts in a food processor and pulse until the hazelnuts are coarsely ground. Transfer to a mixing bowl and stir in the ground almonds and sugar.

In a small pan, gently heat the butter and dark chocolate together until melted. Stir into the nut mixture.

Line a baking sheet with baking parchment over a baking sheet. Spread the chocolate mixture over the baking parchment, making a roughly square or rectangular shape about 5mm thick.

Transfer to the freezer and freeze for about 30 minutes. Remove the brittle from the freezer and, working quickly, chop into about 12 pieces. Use a fish slice to remove the brittle from the tray and place in a freezer-proof plastic container. Return to the freezer as quickly as possible and keep frozen until needed.

Fruit and nut brownies

These amazing brownies are rich in both protein and fibre, are very filling and have just the right amount of sweetness. As the recipe uses coconut flour it does take a while to cook but the results are worth it. They keep for longer than you might expect, up to 7 days in an airtight container.

makes 16   10 mins   1 hour   **83** calories

50g butter, softened, plus extra for greasing
50g raisins
30g cocoa powder
30g stevia
2 tbsp soft dark brown sugar
1 large egg
50g coconut flour
1 tsp baking powder
1 tsp xanthan gum
1 tsp vanilla bean paste
50g cashews, roughly chopped

Low sugar	✓
Protein-rich	✓

Preheat the oven to 180°C/160°C fan/350°F/gas mark 4 and lightly grease a 20cm square cake tin and line the base with baking parchment.

Place the raisins and cocoa in a small bowl and pour over 300ml of boiling water. Stir in and leave to rest while you prepare the rest of the ingredients.

In a large bowl, beat the butter, stevia and brown sugar together until smooth. Beat in the egg.

Add the coconut flour, baking powder, xanthan gum and vanilla bean paste to the batter and mix thoroughly. Pour in the cocoa and raisin mixture and stir again. It will become thicker and gloopier as the coconut flour absorbs the water. Stir in the chopped cashews.

Spoon into the prepared tin and level off the mixture. Bake for approximately 1 hour, or until a skewer inserted into the middle comes out clean. Leave to cool in the tin completely before removing to a chopping board and cutting into 16 equal pieces. Store in a cake tin or individually wrapped for up to 5 days.

Peach melba tray bake

This is one of my favourite low sugar and low-carb cakes. It has a lovely taste and structure.

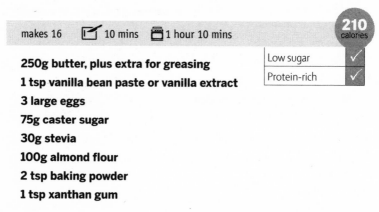

makes 16	10 mins	1 hour 10 mins	210 calories

Low sugar	✓
Protein-rich	✓

250g butter, plus extra for greasing
1 tsp vanilla bean paste or vanilla extract
3 large eggs
75g caster sugar
30g stevia
100g almond flour
2 tsp baking powder
1 tsp xanthan gum

50g ground almonds
3 peaches, peeled, stoned and roughly chopped
100g raspberries
1 tbsp flaked almonds
1 tbsp icing sugar

Preheat the oven to 180°C/160°C fan/350°F/gas mark 4 and grease a small cake tin, about 20cm square.

Heat the butter until just melted in a small pan. Allow to cool slightly before beating in the vanilla and eggs.

In a large bowl, combine the sugar and stevia with the almond flour, baking powder, xanthan gum and ground almonds. Pour in the butter and egg mixture and stir thoroughly.

Pour the gloopy mixture into the prepared tin and level out with the back of a spoon.

Arrange the chopped peaches and raspberries over the top and sprinkle on the flaked almonds.

Cover with foil and bake for 50 minutes before removing the foil and baking for a further 20 minutes. Leave to cool completely in the tin. When cold, transfer to a chopping board, dust over the icing sugar and cut into squares.

Hazelnut and cranberry chocolates

The trick with these lovely treats is to melt the chocolate really, really slowly in the microwave, as this acts as a cheat's way of tempering your chocolate. If you don't your chocolate may 'bloom', resulting in ugly white patches.

makes about 16   10 mins   **53** calories

100g dark chocolate (70% cocoa solids)
½ tsp stevia
20g dried cranberries
30g hazelnuts, halved

Low sugar ✓

Cover a baking sheet with baking parchment or a silicone sheet.

Chop your chocolate into small pieces, at least half the size of the standard 'squares'. Place in a small microwave-safe bowl with the stevia. Microwave on high in very short bursts (no more than 10 seconds), stirring briefly after each burst. When about half the chocolate is molten and you have a pool of molten chocolate with some pieces floating in it, remove from the microwave. Start stirring immediately and keep stirring until every last square of chocolate is melted. The chocolate will be thick and close to setting point so you'll need to work quickly from now on.

Put a teaspoon of chocolate on to the prepared baking sheet and swirl with the back of the spoon to make a circle about the size of a £2 coin. Immediately press about 2 pieces each of hazelnut and cranberries into the chocolate. Repeat until you have about 16 chocolates. Leave in a cool place (but not the fridge) to set. Keep cool.

Fabulous flapjacks

*These squidgy flapjacks are sweetened only with fruit and
a little honey. Jam-packed with good stuff, these flapjacks
should be kept in the fridge to keep them at their best.*

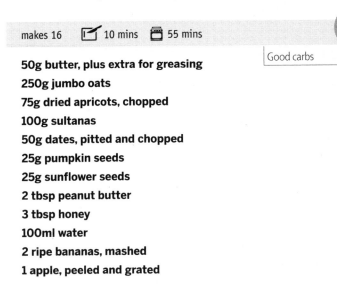

makes 16   10 mins   55 mins   **172** calories

Good carbs ✓

50g butter, plus extra for greasing
250g jumbo oats
75g dried apricots, chopped
100g sultanas
50g dates, pitted and chopped
25g pumpkin seeds
25g sunflower seeds
2 tbsp peanut butter
3 tbsp honey
100ml water
2 ripe bananas, mashed
1 apple, peeled and grated

Preheat oven to 160°C/140°C fan/325°F/gas mark 3 and lightly grease a 20cm square cake tin and line the base with baking parchment.

In a large mixing bowl, mix together the oats, apricots, sultanas, dates and seeds.

In a small non-stick pan, gently heat the butter, peanut butter, honey and water together. When dissolved, stir in the mashed banana and grated apple.

Pour the banana and apple mixture over the oats and stir until everything is combined. Spoon into the cake tin and level with the back of the spoon. Bake for 55 minutes, until turning golden on top. Leave to cool in the tin and then transfer to a chopping board and cut into 16 pieces. Keep in an airtight container in the fridge.

Ginger oat biscuits

A great snacking biscuit that everyone will love. As a cheat's alternative to cheesecake these are delicious topped with a spoonful of Greek yoghurt and some fresh berries.

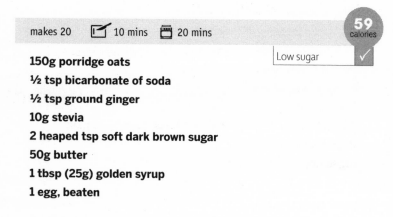

makes 20 ☑ 10 mins 🍲 20 mins

59 calories

Low sugar ✓

150g porridge oats
½ tsp bicarbonate of soda
½ tsp ground ginger
10g stevia
2 heaped tsp soft dark brown sugar
50g butter
1 tbsp (25g) golden syrup
1 egg, beaten

Preheat the oven to 160°C/140°C fan/325°F/gas mark 3.

Place the oats, bicarbonate of soda, ginger, stevia and brown sugar in a large bowl and mix until well combined.

Melt the butter and golden syrup together in the microwave on a low setting. Pour the melted butter into the dry ingredients along with the beaten egg. Mix together into a sticky dough.

Use 2 large sheets of baking parchment or silicone sheets to roll out the dough. Spoon the mixture into the middle of the first sheet. Place the second sheet over the top and roll out into an even rectangle about 3–5mm thick. Carefully peel back the top sheet of paper.

Transfer the dough, still on the bottom sheet of paper to a large baking tray.

Bake in the oven for 15–20 minutes until golden. Leave to cool slightly before cutting into squares and cooling completely on a wire rack.

Honey seed snaps

A simple crunchy snack that everyone will love.

SERVES 12   ⌁ 5 mins   🗄 20 mins

88
calories

100g mixed seeds, such as sesame, sunflower, pumpkin
50g butter
30g honey

Preheat the oven to 190°C/170°C fan/375°F/gas mark 5 and line a small cake tin with baking parchment.

If necessary, chop up any larger seeds as finely as possible.

Heat the butter and honey together in a small pan until the butter has melted and the honey has dissolved. Pour the butter and honey mixture into the prepared baking tray. Rock the tray gently to allow the liquid to spread over the base of the tin.

Sprinkle the seeds over the butter and honey. The idea is to make a thin even layer of seeds. Push any seeds that are sticking above the butter and honey down into the mix with your fingers.

Bake in the oven for 10–12 minutes, until browned. Leave in the tin until cool enough to handle and then transfer to a chopping board. Use a blunt knife to cut it into 12 pieces and then move to a wire rack to cool completely.

Chocolate hazelnut torte

This decadent dessert is good enough to be served at the best dinner parties. Or just when you fancy a delicious treat.

| SERVES 8 | 20 mins | 30 mins | 10 mins | **425** calories |

Low sugar ✓

For the base
150g ground almonds
15g cocoa powder
1 tsp stevia
30g butter, melted, plus extra for greasing

For the filling
250g mascarpone
30g hazelnuts, roughly chopped
20g cocoa
2 tbsp stevia
3 large egg whites

For the topping
50g dark chocolate, broken into pieces
30g butter
3 large egg yolks

1 tsp stevia
20g hazelnuts, halved

Preheat the oven to 210°C/190°C fan/425°F/gas mark 7 and lightly grease a 20cm loose-bottomed cake tin.

To make the base, mix together the ground almonds, cocoa and stevia in a large bowl. Pour in the melted butter and stir to combine. Spoon the mixture into the prepared cake tin and press down firmly with your fingers to make a firm and even base. Bake in the oven for 10 minutes, then leave to cool.

To prepare the filling, mix together the mascarpone, hazelnuts, cocoa and stevia in a bowl. In a separate clean bowl, whisk the egg whites until they form stiff peaks. Spoon a third of the egg whites into the mascarpone and mix well, then fold in the remaining egg whites.

Distribute the filling over the base and refrigerate for about 30 minutes, or freeze for 10 minutes. Remove from the cake tin and place on a serving plate.

To make the topping, place the chocolate and butter in a pan over a low/medium heat and stir until melted. Beat the egg yolks and stevia together in a bowl until slightly thickened and then beat in the melted chocolate and butter. Quickly pour the thick chocolate sauce over the top of the torte, using a knife to even up the topping if necessary. Arrange the hazelnuts over the top and press lightly into the chocolate. Chill in the fridge until ready to serve.

Buttery shortbread

A surprisingly easy and tasty recipe for shortbread using ground almonds.

SERVES 8 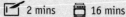 2 mins ▦ 16 mins

250g ground almonds
1 tbsp stevia
100g butter, melted

Preheat the oven to 210°C/190°C fan/425°F/gas mark 7 and lightly butter a 20cm loose-bottomed cake tin.

Mix the ground almonds and stevia in a bowl. Pour in the melted butter and stir to form a dough. Scoop the mixture into the prepared tin and flatten with the back of a spoon. Use a fork to make pinpricks all over the dough.

Bake in the oven for 14–16 minutes, until just starting to turn golden. Cool for a few minutes in the tin before carefully turning out and cutting into wedges.

Recipe Index

Breakfast basics

Simple snacks

Lovely lunches

Speedy suppers

Delicious dinners

Family favourites

Sides and veggies

Puddings

Baking and cakes